Other monographs in the series, Major Problems in Clinical Surgery:

SURGERY OF THE BILIARY TRACT

by

Bjorn Thorbjarnarson, M.D.

Professor of Surgery
Cornell University Medical College;
Acting Chairman and Surgeon-in-Chief
Department of Surgery
New York Hospital – Cornell University
Medical Center

Volume XVI in the Series
MAJOR PROBLEMS IN CLINICAL SURGERY
J. ENGLEBERT DUNPHY
PAUL A. EBERT
Consulting Editors

W. B. Saunders Company, Philadelphia, London, Toronto, 1975

W. B. Saunders Company: West Washington Square
Philadelphia, PA 19105

12 Dyott Street
London, WC1A 1DB

833 Oxford Street
Toronto, Ontario M8Z 5T9, Canada

Surgery of the Biliary Tract   ISBN 0-7216-8858-6

Last digit is the print number: 9   8   7   6   5   4   3   2   1

Foreword

The purpose of this monograph is to elucidate the status of surgery of the biliary tract. Dr. Thorbjarnarson has had extensive experience in diseases of this area and presents the pathophysiology, diagnosis, and treatment in a manner that should be helpful to all involved in surgical practice. The high frequency of diseases of the biliary system makes a thorough understanding of them necessary. Too often the gallbladder and bile ducts are regarded lightly by both internist and surgeon, yet there is no other system so likely to produce chronic and recurrent problems if the initial therapy is incorrect. Dr. Dunphy, who so capably guided the Major Problems in Clinical Surgery through its first fifteen volumes, has over the years stressed the high number of chronic debilitating complications resulting from surgical mismanagement of the biliary system. It is a pleasure, then, for me to introduce my first nomination for the series, one that I hope will be most useful in bringing improvement to our approach to patients with biliary disease.

PAUL A. EBERT, M.D.

Preface

This book is written as a comprehensive approach to the surgical care of biliary tract disease in adult life. It is a very personal approach but I have tried to eliminate quirks of the sort that many of us are personally fond of but that really do not help the vast number of surgeons doing biliary surgery. Gadgetry dictated by individual tastes and idiosyncrasies usually is not applicable to our generation of surgeons as a whole. Since 300,000 to 400,000 cholecystectomies are done each year in the United States, it is obvious that these operations are done in most hospitals and by most general surgeons. The approach to the problem thus should be as simple as possible if the largest number of patients are to receive the greatest possible benefit.

The results of biliary tract surgery when performed by the properly trained surgeon utilizing well founded principles are very good at present and have never been better. This does not mean that there is not room for improvement, and this improvement is bound to come, particularly in the realm of possible dissolution of gallstones without surgery, the diagnosis of jaundice through retrograde cholangiography and improved ways of finding common duct stones intraoperatively.

No one reading this book will fail to see how the work and spirit of Dr. Frank Glenn has influenced its making. His influence as my teacher and the leader of the past and present generation of biliary tract surgeons will be noted for years to come.

My thanks also to Dr. Kevin Morrissey for the chapter on physiology and biochemistry of the system, and to Dr. Paul Ebert for his encouragement in the writing of this book.

New York
June 1st, 1975

Contents

Chapter One

HISTORY OF BILIARY TRACT SURGERY

The history of biliary tract operations goes back to the Middle Ages or earlier, although documentation of early experiments is difficult. Fabricius Hildaneus was supposed to have removed gallstones from the gallbladder in the year 1618, but it is not stated whether the operation was performed on a living human being.[1] In the 17th century animal experiments were frequently undertaken. In 1667 the gallbladder was removed from a dog by Teckop in Leiden, Holland. The first known suggestion to remove gallstones from human beings came from J. L. Petit, but it apparently did not create any enthusiasm and was not undertaken. A. G. Richter suggested that a pus-filled gallbladder might be emptied through a trocar through the abdominal wall. In 1859 Thudichum suggested that a cholecystostomy could be done in two stages — first by creating adhesions between the gallbladder and the abdominal wall, and by incising and draining the gallbladder without danger of spilling bile into the peritoneal cavity. This was not carried out either, as far as is known.

In 1867 John Bobbs in Indianapolis carried out the first documented cholecystostomy.[1, 2] This was not a planned cholecystostomy, however, but rather an operation for a tumor in the abdomen. When the tumor was opened, large numbers of gallstones emerged unexpectedly. In 1882 König performed an operation on the gallbladder by cholecystotomy in two stages. Before König's operation, however, the first known planned operation on the biliary tree was done in 1878 by J. Marion Sims, an American surgeon who at that time was practicing in France.[3] Dr. Sims did a cholecystostomy on a woman who was suffering long-standing jaundice and gallbladder colic. The operation itself was successful and the woman was greatly relieved.

1

However, she died ten days later from massive internal hemorrhage probably brought on by lack of vitamin K absorption from the intestine and prolonged prothrombin time. The reason for this was not evident at that time.

In 1882 Langenbuch in Germany initiated modern surgery of the biliary tree by removing the gallbladder in its entirety, together with the stones contained within it. Langenbuch thought that gallstones were formed in the gallbladder and that only removal of the gallbladder itself would prevent reformation of the stones. Following Langenbuch's operation progress was rapid, and soon thereafter the common bile duct was opened surgically and stones retrieved from the common duct. Courvoisier was one of the first surgeons to open the common duct for removal of stones. It should be mentioned that prior to surgical intervention for biliary tract disease, the fate of persons with gallstones was a rather sorry one. The only hope for the sufferers of common duct obstruction from stones or acute purulent infection from the gallbladder was that fistulas from the outside of the internal organs would form, permitting stones to be extruded either into the intestine or to the outside. This would create a biliary fistula with decompression of the biliary system and consequent relief of jaundice or septic infection.

REFERENCES

1. Kleinschmidt, O.: Operative Chirurgie. Berlin, Springer-Verlag, 1948, p. 1234.
2. Glen, F., and Grafe, W. F.: Historical events in biliary tract surgery. Arch. Surg. 93:848, 1966.
3. Sims, J. M.: Remarks on cholecystostomy in dropsy of the gallbladder. Br. Med. J. June 8, 1879, p. 811.

Chapter Two

DIAGNOSIS OF BILIARY TRACT DISEASE

THE DIFFERENTIAL DIAGNOSIS OF JAUNDICE[1]

Jaundice is caused by the accumulation of bile pigment bilirubin in the blood. The accumulation of bile pigments may result from over-production, i.e., excessive breakdown of red blood cells in the spleen, from interference with the excretion of bilirubin by the liver, or from blockage of the bile after it leaves the liver, i.e, obstruction in the ductal system. I prefer to think in terms of prehepatic, hepatic, and posthepatic jaundice. As surgeons we are called upon to correct some prehepatic and posthepatic jaundice by surgery, and we must be able to weed out the patients with hepatic jaundice, since surgery is not likely to be helpful except for diagnostic purposes.

Prehepatic Jaundice

Prehepatic jaundice is usually caused by excessive hemolysis of the red cells by the reticuloendothelial system and is found in both inherited and acquired hemolytic anemias. It may be involved in absorption of large hematomas or found in patients with sepsis. This type of jaundice, also called retention jaundice, is caused by an overload of unconjugated bilirubin. It is usually easily diagnosed by a characteristic history, normal liver function tests, the absence of urobilinogen in the urine, and normal-colored stools. Visualization of

3

the biliary tree is possible by oral or intravenous administration of iodized preparations.

Hepatic Jaundice

Jaundice caused by primary damage to the liver cell constitutes one of the most common types of jaundice. The bilirubin in the blood is of both the conjugated and unconjugated types: the inability of the damaged hepatic cells to accept all the breakdown products of the hemoglobin causes the presence of the unconjugated type; the presence of a significant conjugated portion (regurgitation jaundice) is caused by failure of the hepatic cell to excrete bilirubin after conjuga-

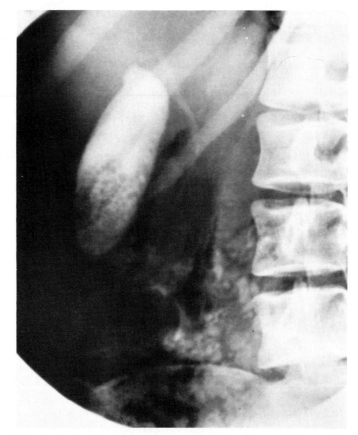

Figure 2–1 A cholecystogram from a jaundiced patient with hemolytic anemia. In spite of the jaundice the liver function is normal, and the gallbladder, containing multiple small stones, is well visualized. A small part of the common bile duct is also seen and is the normal size. Only in hemolytic jaundice, in which liver function is normal, does visualization of the biliary tree occur.

tion. Typically this is the jaundice of viral hepatitis, but it also includes liver damage from other causes — drugs, alcohol, and serum hepatitis. Usually there is evidence of relatively increased amounts of unconjugated bilirubin in the blood; the liver enzymes, SGOT and SGPT, are elevated in the 600 to 700 range or over; alkaline phosphatase is normal or only slightly elevated; the prothrombin time is prolonged and responds poorly to vitamin K; the stool contains bile; and there is urobilinogen in the urine.

Posthepatic Jaundice

Posthepatic jaundice, the jaundice with which surgeons are primarily involved, is of the same nature as the hepatic type of jaundice, except that in the beginning the bilirubin is mainly or solely of the conjugated type, having passed through the liver cell and then been regurgitated because of the obstruction in the bile duct. This is the jaundice caused by tumors, stones, or strictures in the extrahepatic ductal system. The history is usually typical: either a patient has pain and fever of biliary colic preceding the jaundice, or an otherwise healthy person notices dark urine, itching, and scleral icterus caused by the malignant tumor of the extrahepatic duct system. Typically the liver function tests are normal or only slightly abnormal in the beginning, except for an elevated alkaline phosphatase. This picture predominates in carcinomatous obstruction of the pancreas or bile duct. Bile duct obstruction caused by a common duct stone or acute cholecystitis may show different results, since the cholangitis accompanying the obstruction may cause early damage to the liver cells, resulting in high levels of liver enzymes with only slightly increased alkaline phosphatase. In these patients serial observations of blood tests are important; usually within a week the obstructive nature of the inflammatory illness is clearly evident.

Investigation of the Patient with Jaundice

Taking the History

The taking of a history from a patient with jaundice may often provide the basis for a tentative diagnosis. A history of exposure to hepatotoxic agents (ingestion of drugs known to be hepatotoxic, including alcohol, drug habit), transfusions, anemia, or familial jaundice may be of importance. Previous symptoms of cholelithiasis or known cholelithiasis may support a diagnosis of obstruction. The painless jaundice of malignancy occurring in an otherwise healthy person is also typical.

Physical Examination

Together with the history, the physical examination often clinches the diagnosis. The most accurate and valuable finding is a Courvoisier's gallbladder. The finding of a distended, nontender gallbladder with a history of painless jaundice establishes the diagnosis of a carcinomatous obstruction distal to the cystic duct and is the only physical finding to establish a diagnosis in jaundice. Other important findings are the cholesterol skin deposits and extensive scratch marks of biliary cirrhosis. The finding of an enlarged spleen may be evidence of primary hepatocellular disease, but it also may indicate carcinoma of the body of the pancreas blocking the splenic vein. In either case the history will usually confirm the correct diagnosis. Spider angiomas with gynecomastia, testicular atrophy, and palmar erythema should indicate primary liver cell disease, and a history of excessive alcohol intake would support that diagnosis. Ascites usually indicates primary liver cell disease and cirrhosis, but it may also occur in carcinoma of the pancreas and biliary tree.

For the surgeon the history and physical examination may indicate surgical disease or may point to the necessity for particularly careful evaluation. The evidence of surgical disease is found primarily in the patient with painless jaundice and palpable gallbladder or with a history of gallbladder disease with stones, leading to an acute attack of pain with jaundice following. Careful evaluation must be made of the young patient with considerable prodromata before the onset of jaundice, of the patient with ascites or splenomegaly or both, of the patient with a drug habit, and of the alcoholic with the usual signs of cirrhosis.

Clinical Tests on Patients with Jaundice

There are many blood tests that assist the surgeon in the differential diagnosis of nonobstructive and obstructive jaundice. These tests are not specific, however, but they do help in separating the patients into the broad groups. The tests indicate liver function, liver cell obstruction, and bile regurgitation. The test that best indicates liver function is the prothrombin time, and it is quite valuable, particularly when also evaluated in response to vitamin K administration. Vitamin K is fat-soluble and is only absorbed from the intestines in the presence of bile. Prothrombin is made in the liver and can only be produced adequately in the presence of healthy liver cells and vitamin K. The prothrombin time is affected earlier in liver damage than in vitamin K deficiency and thus becomes abnormal sooner in parenchymatous or hepatocellular diseases than in pure biliary obstruction. When vitamin K is given intramuscularly, there is usually a poor response in the prothrombin time in the presence of heptocellular disease but a prompt response when primary extra-hepatic obstruction exists. Determination of serum transaminase level, SGOT and SGPT, evaluates the magnitude of liver cell de-struction. Thus these values tend to be elevated (over 600 to 700) in hepatocellular disease (hepatitis) and low or normal in primary obstruction. In the early phases of obstructive jaundice, most often caused by stones but sometimes by carcinoma, the initial insult of complete obstruction, together with infection and cholangitis, is enough to cause a significant rise in the transaminase levels, even up to levels suggestive of hepatitis. As time goes by, however, these values decrease, and the reverse occurs in the alkaline phosphatase levels. The serum alkaline phosphatase or the 5-nucleotidase levels are sensitive indicators of bile duct obstruction and show an early and predominant rise. These values are increased in obstruction at the level of the minor bile duct and when obstruction is limited to one hepatic duct. Thus in tumor obstruction of one hepatic duct or with liver metastases, alkaline phosphatase is elevated long before jaundice occurs.

Serum cholesterol is usually significantly elevated in obstructive jaundice and particularly so in primary biliary cirrhosis. The serum protein level alters in chronic and long-standing liver disease; the globulin fraction increases and ultimately may reverse its normal relationship to the serum albumin fraction.

Special Tests in the Differential Diagnosis of Jaundice

Among the tests used for differential diagnosis is the cortisone suppression test, in which jaundice diminishes and perhaps dis-appears when hepatocellular damage is responsible. Unfortunately this test is not altogether reliable, since decrease in jaundice may also be seen when primary obstruction exists. The ^{131}I rose bengal excre-tion test relies on the liver to clear the rose bengal from the blood-stream and excrete it into the duodenum, where it may be seen on scanning, giving evidence of patency of the extrahepatic ductal sys-tem. This test is not altogether reliable, since incomplete obstruction gives false information. A technetium scan of the liver itself is helpful in obscure cases, particularly when the jaundice is caused by a liver abscess. It is less reliable in jaundice caused by tumor metastases. Hepatic angiography becomes useful in delineating masses within the liver and may also indicate the presence of cirrhosis. Radiographic examination of the upper gastrointestinal tract is often helpful in evaluation of the patient with jaundice. The presence of esophageal varices in connection with jaundice would indicate primary intrahepatic obstruction, whereas a filling defect in the duodenum may show an ampullar or duodenal carcinoma. An enlarged gallbladder or common duct often produces an impression on the duodenum, indicating the obstructive nature of the jaundice.

Liver Biopsy

A percutaneous biopsy of the liver is indicated in jaundice when the total findings indicate that hepatocellular damage rather than extrahepatic obstruction is the cause. For the biopsy to be safely performed, the prothrombin time must be reasonably normal, and there should be no evidence of portal hypertension. The biopsy may provide the final proof for the diagnosis of hepatitis or fatty degeneration as the cause of jaundice, but in the case of cholestatic intrahepatic disease due to drugs or primary cirrhosis, the results may be equivocal and not decisive for diagnosis. Liver biopsy is dangerous when extrahepatic obstruction exists, since bile under pressure may escape into the peritoneal cavity and cause rapid and sometimes fatal peritonitis unless immediate surgical decompression is undertaken.

In most patients the nature of the jaundice, obstructive or not, may be established with a few days of investigation. A few patients present a confusing picture. This is particularly true in cases of intrahepatic cholestasis from drugs or in some instances of extrahepatic obstruction associated with a degree of cholangitis. In these patients a prolonged period of observation—two to three weeks—may be needed to establish a diagnosis; during this time changes in liver chemistry indicating cellular disease or extrahepatic obstruction are followed. In even fewer instances the definitive diagnosis cannot be made without further investigation, often by laparotomy, but more and more by percutaneous cholangiography or retrograde cholangiography through the duodenoscope.

RADIOGRAPHIC EXAMINATION OF THE BILIARY TRACT

Cholecystography has been practiced since 1924 when Graham and Cole introduced its practical application. Today it is a remarkably simple and effective way of demonstrating disease of the gallbladder.

Various compounds of iodinated contrast agents have been used, but the one commonly in use now and discussed here is iopanoic acid (Telepaque). The usual dose of Telepaque is 3 g (6 tablets) taken the night before. In order for the test to be reliable, some criteria have to be fulfilled. First of all the patient must take the tablets, and this can usually be seen on the initial scout film of the abdomen, since some of the material usually remains in the intestinal tract. The patient must also be able to retain the tablets. Vomiting from organic or inorganic causes is a common reason for nonvisualization. The tablet must not produce diarrhea, since the material may then be passed through the intestinal tract without absorption. The patient's liver function must be adequate for excretion of the material into the bile ducts. Usually a cholecystogram will be unsuccessful when serum bilirubin is above 2 mg per 100 ml or BSP reaction is greater than 40 per cent.[2] In spite of attention to these criteria, it is recognized that additional contrast material is needed by some patients for adequate visualization of the gallbladder. When the first dose does not produce adequate visualization of the gallbladder, a second dose (6 tablets) is given within 48 hours of the first study, and the x-rays are repeated. A study performed at the New York Hospital of 5000 patients examined by cholecystography from 1970 to 1972 revealed the following result.[3] Seventy-five per cent of the gallbladders on the first examination were adequately opacified for establishment of diagnosis. Twenty-five per cent were inadequately opacified and required administration of a second dose. After the second dose, 67 per cent were adequately opacified for diagnosis. Of these, 80 per cent were found to be normal. Twenty per cent were found diseased, the great majority with calculi but a few with adenomyomas, cholesterosis, or Aschoff-Rokitansky sinuses. At the conclusion of the second-dose study, there remained 413 patients whose gallbladders still failed to opacify adequately for diagnosis. A close examination of these remaining patients revealed the following reasons for failure of the gallbladder to visualize. Forty-four patients were discovered to have liver disease of sufficient magnitude to prevent excretion. Seventeen were found already to have had their gallbladders removed. In some instances this was unknown to the patient; in other instances the examination had been ordered inadvertently. Five patients had pyloric obstruction, one had previously undergone a cholecystojejunostomy, and in one instance the patient had never taken the Telepaque. There remained 345 patients in whom the gallbladder failed to opacify after the second dose without known extrinsic causes. Of these patients, 193 did not have surgery performed for various reasons, and the condition of their gallbladders is still unknown. Of the 152 patients who underwent surgery, all were found to have diseased gallbladders: 135 had calculi, three had carcinoma of the gallbladder with calculi, seven had acute cholecystitis, and the rest had chronic cholecystitis, with one patient suffering from cholangiocarcinoma invading the gallbladder. The study reported here indicates how very reliable the one- or two-dose cholecystogram can be when it is properly performed and when the pitfalls associated with nonvisualization are taken into account. The addition of intravenous cholangiography for further clarification of gallbladder disease may be confusing and not too rewarding except as it confirms cystic duct obstruction. There were 80 IVC's performed in the above group following nonvisualization of the gallbladder after two doses of Telepaque. In 51 of these, nonvisualization was confirmed. In 14 patients the gallbladder filled and appeared normal, whereas at operation all 14 were found to have diseased gallbladders (12 had calculi). In 15 patients the gallbladder filled and stones were diagnosed. The filling of the gallbladder in these instances by the IVC therefore gave erroneous information. The opacification of the gallbladder on the oral studies is based on the concentrating ability of the gallbladder. The contrast material used for IVC is already in high concentration when it leaves the liver and thus will opacify a gallbladder that has lost its concentrating ability. The opacification, however, is commonly inadequate for demonstrating stones within the gallbladder. The use of IVC for the diagnosis of chronic gallbladder disease therefore appears to have limited value and sometimes to give erroneous results.

CHOLANGIOGRAPHY

The diagnosis of biliary tree diseases improved greatly with the advent of oral cholecystography in the 1920s and intravenous cholangiography in the 1940s. Through these procedures we can now delineate the biliary tree in patients in whom the excretory function of the liver is still adequate and, in the case of oral cholecystography, in those in whom absorption of the medium takes place in the intestinal tract. Visualization of the biliary tree by these methods becomes impossible when the excretory function of the liver fails, and in practice these tests are useless in the presence of serum bilirubin levels of 2 to 3 mg per 100 ml, except when caused by hemolysis.

Percutaneous Cholangiography

A surgeon faced with a jaundiced patient must first decide whether the cause is parenchymal and falls into the realm of hepatitis or cirrhosis, or whether an extrahepatic obstruction exists that will require surgery. Physical examination will often furnish the answer.

Palpation of a distended Courvoisier's gallbladder is as important a finding as any blood test or x-ray and indicates the presence of tumor obstruction distal to the cystic duct.

A wide range of blood tests is available to separate parenchymal from obstructive jaundice. Occasionally acute liver damage may occur due to obstruction from tumor, and levels of serum glutamic and serum glutamic pyruvic transaminase may rise significantly, but the rise is short-lived and overshadowed by an elevated alkaline phosphatase. The same may be said about obstruction due to calculous disease. Usually, by virtue of clinical examination and tests, the picture becomes clear and a differential diagnosis can be made. The surgeon is then left with a small number of patients in whom the differential diagnosis between obstructive and nonobstructive jaundice cannot be made, and a fairly large group of patients in whom obstructive jaundice can be demonstrated but the site or level of obstruction remains unknown until the time of operation.

Percutaneous transhepatic cholangiography is successful in delineating the bile duct in a high percentage (85 per cent) of patients with obstructive jaundice and in a significantly lower percentage (less than 50 per cent) of patients with parenchymal jaundice. The procedure should not be used as a shortcut in the diagnosis of jaundice; rather, it should be used after all the conventional methods have been exhausted, and then only with the patient prepared for surgery the same day. The procedure is not without discomfort, and the patient needs to be sedated beforehand; 100 mg each of Demerol and phenobarbital is usually sufficient for adults. When normal bile ducts are demonstrated, surgery of course need not be performed, since obstruction has been ruled out and the cause of the jaundice located in the liver parenchyma. When the cholangiogram is unsuccessful, as happens in up to 15 per cent of patients with extrahepatic obstruction, operation should be carried out anyway and the cause of jaundice located by conventional means during operation. To assume that an unsuccessful cholangiogram rules out obstructive jaundice is fallacious and dangerous, since bile peritonitis may well result.

Aside from occasionally diagnosing cases of hepatitis and thus saving patients from surgery, the greatest advantage of percutaneous cholangiography is the localization of obstructive lesions in the hepatic duct or at the bifurcation of the hepatic duct. During laparotomy for jaundice, the surgeon is confused by a normal bladder and common bile duct. In the absence of the cholangiogram he may reason that the patient indeed has parenchymal liver disease and perform no more than a liver biopsy. If the surgeon opens the normal common duct and finds an obstruction proximally, either by probing or by x-ray, he does not know the proximal extent of the lesion encountered and thus is hampered in selecting a procedure for even a palliative decompression.

It is indeed true that at this point an intraoperative transhepatic cholangiogram may be done, but usually the quality of portable cholangiograms leaves something to be desired.

A second group of patients in whom percutaneous cholangiography is most helpful is composed of those who have iatrogenic strictures of the bile ducts. Operations in these instances are usually difficult and test the surgeon, since the procedure commonly follows a cholecystectomy by only a few days or weeks. Accurate preoperative localization of the stricture saves the surgeon from a time-consuming search for the proximal bile duct.

The configuration of the cholangiogram in cases of tumor may be most informative as to the anatomic origin of tumors and thus aid the surgeon in his decision as to type of surgery to be performed. Often the cystic duct and gallbladder are visualized when the tumor obstruction is below the level of the cystic duct. Failure of the gallbladder to fill should alert the surgeon to the possibility that a cholecystoenterostomy might not be the procedure of choice for biliary decompression.

The risks of percutaneous cholangiography are substantial and should not be ignored. Spillage of bile occurs almost always; significant bleeding from the liver substance occurs rarely. Both these complications usually are handled promptly and easily during the laparotomy that should always follow, except when normal bile ducts are demonstrated. Bleeding is apt to occur when there is significant prolongation of the prothrombin time, and the procedure should then be avoided. Sepsis and infection may occur during the procedure, since injection of arteries and veins is common.

Thus cholangiography should be avoided in the presence of frank cholangitis and infection. Properly performed and cautiously applied, the procedure is of great help to the biliary tract surgeon, and it should remain an integral part of his armamentarium in the evaluation and surgery of jaundice.

Retrograde Cholangiography

In the last few years it has become possible to visualize and even cannulate the ampulla of Vater through the flexible duodenoscope.[8,9] Injection of contrast material then makes it possible to visualize the bile ducts, even in the presence of jaundice. Obviously this is an ideal procedure for eliminating surgery as a diagnostic procedure in persons with jaundice of hepatic origin, particularly when the bile ducts are normal in size and thus are difficult to delineate by transhepatic cholangiography. The procedure requires expertise and is only successful in the hands of highly trained persons. Complications may occur, and when biliary obstruction is suspected, it is well to plan surgical intervention on the same day as the cannulation, since sepsis and cholangitis may result from injection of material into an obstructed biliary system. The advantages of this examination, however, clearly outweigh the possible complications. Transduodenal cannulation will not supplant transhepatic cholangiography, since it often will show only the distal part of an obstructing lesion, whereas the transhepatic cholangiogram shows the proximal end of the lesion along with the intrahepatic ductal system and thus indicates to the surgeon types of decompression procedures applicable to the individual patient.

REFERENCES

1. Zimmerman, H. J.: The differential diagnosis of jaundice. Med. Clin. North Am. 52:1417, 1968.
2. Kreel, L.: Radiology of the biliary system. Clinics in Gastroenterology 2:185, 1973.
3. Mujahed, Z.: Personal communication.
4. Burkhardt, H., and Muller, W.: Versuche uber die Punktion der Gallenblase und Ihre Rontgendarstellung. Dtsch. Z. Chir. 161–162:168–197, 1921.
5. Glenn, F., Evans, J. A., Mujahed, Z., and Thorbjarnarson, B.: Percutaneous transhepatic cholangiography. Ann. Surg. 156:451, 1962.
6. Thorbjarnarson, B.: Mujahed, Z., and Glenn, F.: Percutaneous transhepatic cholangiography. Ann. Surg. 165:33, 1967.
7. Myers, R. N., Deaver, J. M., Haupt, G. J., and Birkhead, N. C.: Percutaneous transhepatic cholangiography and cinecholangiography. Arch. Surg. 97:51, 1968.
8. Cotton, P. B.: Cannulation of the papilla of Vater by endoscopy and retrograde cholangiopancreatography (ERCP). Gut 13:1014, 1972.
9. Dickinson, P. B., Belsito, A. A., and Cramer, G. G.: Diagnostic value of endoscopic cholangiopancreatography. J.A.M.A. 225:944, 1973.

Chapter Three

CURRENT CONCEPTS OF GALLSTONE FORMATION

Kevin P. Morrissey

The purpose of this chapter is to present an overview of current concepts and research efforts concerning the pathogenesis of cholesterol gallstones and then to discuss the recent attempts to dissolve gallstones, based on our present understanding of the factors involved in their formation.

During the past decade, the advances in our knowledge of hepatobiliary tract metabolism have been so rapid and extensive that a thorough evaluation of gallstone formation in a particular individual might encompass the following broad areas: (a) the chemical composition of the bile secreted by the liver; (b) the role of the gallbladder in altering the physiochemical state of hepatic bile flowing into it; and (c) genetic, environmental, and metabolic considerations affecting the liver and gallbladder function. These broad areas will be reviewed, with an attempt to indicate their individual significance, interactions, and net effects on stone formation and dissolution.

CHEMICAL COMPOSITION OF BILE

Lithogenic Bile

The keynote of cholesterol gallstone formation is precipitation of cholesterol from the mixed micelle, or small soluble aggregate of cholesterol, bile salt, and lecithin. It is now barely seven years since

Small and his co-workers here and abroad began to publish a continuing series of major contributions to the physiochemical basis of bile and cholesterol gallstone formation.[1-3] Working with in vitro model systems of bile salts, lecithin, and cholesterol in varying proportions in water, he recognized that cholesterol solubility in an aqueous system such as bile is a function of the relative and not the absolute concentrations of constituents in the system. Solubility limits of cholesterol in any simulated or natural bile specimen could be identified as a point on a triangular phase diagram representing the relative percentage of bile salts, phospholipids, and cholesterol. A "line" of cholesterol solubility could be calculated for phase diagram plots, based on the empirical observation that all test bile solutions plotted beneath it "in the micellar zone" maintain cholesterol in micellar solution; and all solutions plotted above it "outside the micellar zone" are supersaturated with respect to cholesterol and, when allowed to equilibrate, precipitate out crystalline cholesterol.

The early clinical correlations based on this tool for the quantitative characterization of cholesterol solubility in bile produced encouraging but mixed results.[4-8] Bile from patients with gallstones was found to be consistently supersaturated with respect to cholesterol and was considered abnormal or "lithogenic," whereas bile from patients without stones appeared to be unsaturated with respect to cholesterol and, falling within the line of micellar solubility, was considered normal or "nonlithogenic." Further support for this terminology came from a study of Southwest American Indians, who have a very high incidence of cholelithiasis. Then followed reports of gallstone patients having saturation of hepatic as well as gallbladder bile with cholesterol and of apparently healthy people without gallstones who also had lithogenic bile. This suggested that (a) the liver rather than the gallbladder was the source of lithogenic bile; and (b) pregallstone disease could be identified. It also suggested that studies of predisposing genetic and metabolic defects, as well as means for gallstone prophylaxis, might be very productive.

Subsequent studies by Small and many other investigators confirmed, challenged, and modified research methodology, data, and interpretation of the early investigations. Reports of "normal" bile in patients with gallstones and "lithogenic" bile in patients undergoing surgery for unrelated conditions[9] were followed by observations in human beings[10] and baboons[11] that early morning or fasting hepatic bile specimens were invariably supersaturated with cholesterol. In baboons cholesterol-supersaturated hepatic bile was rapidly converted to cholesterol-unsaturated bile by instillation of gallbladder bile into the ileum—the equivalent of gallbladder contraction following a meal. These observations challenged the concept that fasting or supersaturated hepatic bile was really lithogenic, i.e., destined to precipitate out cholesterol. Dam and Hegardt,[9] carrying on studies of dietary induction of gallstones in hamsters, had derived different solubility limits for plotting their own data, and in attempting to apply their criteria to Small's data and that of others, they reclassified many bile samples as being unsaturated rather than supersaturated. Similar criticisms of the original phase diagram method of plotting cholesterol solubility were raised by Holzbach[7] and others[12-14] as each investigator's variable techniques derived a different "line" delineating the limits of cholesterol solubility. The dispute over whose "line" to use has quieted as investigators in the field began to understand the assumptions of each method and, more importantly, that bile composition in patients with or without gallstones is subject to many factors altering it, so that other criteria must be applied in deciding whether a particular subject's bile is truly lithogenic.

In addition to questioning the concept of "abnormal" bile, many investigators have challenged the suggestion that the liver and not the gallbladder is primarily responsible for gallstone formation.[15-17] Recent studies disputing this are covered in the next section. The important point here is that the clinical and experimental exceptions to the basically valid insight of Small regarding chemical criteria for cholesterol solubility in bile stimulated many investigators to study areas apart from the chemical composition of bile for predisposing genetic and metabolic factors, as well as facilitating and limiting cofactors that would cause cholesterol precipitation from an apparently normal individual's occasionally lithogenic bile.

While some investigators' reactions to a revolutionary hypothesis of gallstone formation were to challenge methodology and look for other hypotheses, other investigators chose to dissect the elements of the hypothesis by a more comprehensive investigation of cholesterol, bile salt, and lecithin metabolism and their interactions. Again, Dr. Small had suggested that if a relative excess of cholesterol to bile salt and lecithin existed in bile, it was possibly due to a primary defect in bile or lecithin metabolism that caused insufficient secretion in bile to solubilize the cholesterol present, or conversely, that a primary defect was present in cholesterol metabolism causing excess secretion of it in bile. Defective bile salt and lecithin metabolism will be considered first.

Bile Salts

Decreased bile salt secretion by the liver suggested a deficit in the total pool of bile salts in the enterohepatic circulation. Since 95 to 98 per cent of the bile salts are contained within a normal enterohepatic circulation and techniques for measurement of their pools were known, it remained for Drs. Vlahcevic, Bell, and Swell to show that cholate, and particularly chenodeoxycholate, pool size was decreased in patients with gallstones.[18] Further studies revealed that the cholelithiasis-prone Southwest American Indians have a remarkably low bile salt pool, while the African nomadic Masai tribesmen, in whom gallstones are quite rare, demonstrated the converse finding, i.e., a bile salt pool two to three times normal size.[19-20]

As with the exceptions to the lithogenic bile hypothesis, later studies of different or less homogeneous populations revealed instances of cholelithiasis with normal or even high total bile salt pools, as well as no cholelithiasis in patients with low pools.[21] Nevertheless, the possible significance of decreased bile salt pool size was immediately recognized and has led to the now clinically successful attempts to alter hepatic bile composition in favor of cholesterol solubility and to dissolve gallstones by means of bile salt feeding.[22] The role of bile salt feeding and pool size manipulation will be discussed later.

Phospholipids

The role of phospholipids in cholesterol lithogenesis has received less attention from investigators than that given to bile salts and cholesterol. However, it is increasingly evident, as emphasized in the work of Swell and Tompkins in this country[23-24] and Schersten in Sweden,[25] that successful attempts to analyze or therapeutically manipulate the lithogenic potential of bile must take into account the solubilizing capacity, hepatic synthesis, biliary excretion, metabolism, and intestinal absorption of lecithin.

The synergistic effect of lecithin on the capacity of bile salts to solubilize cholesterol was shown by Isaksson 20 years ago[26] and has been repeatedly demonstrated in the last few years.[23,27] Unlike the bile salts, which are largely conserved and recycled enterohepatically, lecithin and its metabolites are not reabsorbed to a significant degree, and lecithin synthesis in the liver accounts for the majority of the biliary lecithin pool. The importance of this lies in the regulation of lecithin synthesis in the liver and lecithin secretion rate in bile, both of which are tied to bile salt secretion in a direct but not linear relationship.[28,29] Thus, prolonged interruption of the enterohepatic circulation, as in bile stasis in the gallbladder, may result in a marked drop in bile salt recirculation to the liver, with a concomitant decrease in bile salt–stimulated lecithin synthesis. The combination of low bile salt and lecithin excretion into bile can result in a marked reduction of the bile's solubilizing capacity for cholesterol. Schersten has further shown that a direct linear relationship exists between bile salt and cholesterol excretion at bile acid secretion rates above 5 micromoles per minute, but below that level there are completely independent secretion rates of bile acid and cholesterol.[25] Thus, at low flow rates of bile salt, cholesterol secretion does not fall off, and the ratio between cholesterol and lecithin increases rapidly, resulting in bile supersaturated with cholesterol.

These physiologic studies have many exciting recent clinical correlations. Patients with gallstones do often have low biliary phospholipid excretion and decreased lecithin concentration in gallbladder bile, and may also have hypertriglyceridemia.[30, 31] Patients have been described having a combination of gallstones, prebeta-hyperlipoproteinemia, and suggestive evidence for a reduced capacity for hepatic lecithin synthesis.[25] Others have been reported with serum lipoprotein disorders and hypertriglyceridemia.[25, 31] Most exciting are the reports of Tompkins[32] and Bell,[31] who have induced the return of electrophoretic patterns and elevated triglyceride levels to normal by means of lecithin feeding and chenodeoxycholic acid feeding, respectively. The role of lecithin feeding to dissolve gallstones will also be discussed later.

Cholesterol

Cholesterol synthesis and deposition occurs in many tissues throughout the body, but its excretion in the human occurs principally via the hepatobiliary tract and intestine in the form of cholesterol metabolites, the bile acids, and neutral sterols. Unlike the bile salts which are synthesized, contained within, and largely conserved by the enterohepatic circulation, biliary cholesterol derives from dietary ingestion, intestinal absorption, hepatic and small intestinal synthesis, and, to a lesser degree, synthesis in almost all other body tissues. In addition, biliary cholesterol exchanges, at different rates, with the circulatory and tissue compartments outside the enterohepatic circulation. This accounts for the considerable difficulty in characterizing normal, let alone abnormal, cholesterol metabolism in man. Nevertheless, much has been learned recently about cholesterol-bile acid interactions with reference to cholelithiasis.[33-37] The present discussion will be limited to the consideration that abnormal or physiologically altered cholesterol metabolism may contribute to stone formation.

A major breakthrough has occurred within the past three years, namely the development by Grundy of a technique to directly measure hourly biliary lipid secretion in healthy, unoperated, awake subjects.[38] He has found that Indians as a group and many Caucasian women, particularly obese women, have significantly increased secretion of biliary cholesterol and decreased bile salt output, in contrast to Caucasians in general and women or nonobese subjects without gallstones.[33, 39] These findings constitute strong evidence that, at least in some racial populations or individuals, lithogenic bile results from an absolute rather than a relative increase in biliary cholesterol secretion and concentration. The explanations for this increased cholesterol and decreased bile salt secretion are not yet clear, but there is suggestive evidence for a defect in a 7α-hydroxylase-mediated conversion of cholesterol to bile salts.[40] Other rate-limiting enzyme defects or metabolic variables may also account for excessive secretion of biliary cholesterol; it is too early to know the ranges, prevalence, or ultimate significance of cholesterol hypersecretion in man. Many patients with gallstones are not obese or appear to have decreased bile salt pools without increased biliary cholesterol. Also, the conflicting reports of cessation or persistence of cholesterol supersaturation in hepatic bile following cholecystectomy suggest that relative as well as absolute hypersecretion of cholesterol in bile occurs and, depending on the cause, may or may not be significantly altered by cholecystectomy.[41-46]

Another explanation for relative cholesterol hypersecretion in bile is the occurrence of a diurnal variation in hepatic cholesterol secretion.[10] Using the same technique for direct measurement of biliary lipids, Metzger and Grundy found that, in the fasting state, although bile salt and phospholipid secretion in bile drop off markedly as bile is sequestered in the gallbladder, cholesterol secretion in bile continues, especially at low flow rates, independent of bile salt secretion, and renders bile progressively more lithogenic as the fasting state is prolonged. If the fasting state is terminated by a meal or the gallbladder is otherwise stimulated to empty, bile salt and phospholipid secretion in bile increases rapidly and brings cholesterol concentration back into a relatively unsaturated state. This diurnal variation in cholesterol secretion can be detected even if fasting is prolonged; it also has been found by other investigators to have an enzymatic counterpart in the diurnal variation of HMG-CoA reductase, which is an important regulator of hepatic cholesterol synthesis.[47] In addition, diurnal variation in cholesterol secretion occurs in all individuals, including obese women and Indians with gallstones who already have another mechanism contributing to absolute cholesterol hypersecretion. These findings help to explain the prior conflicting reports in which lithogenic bile was found in many people whether or not they had gallstones.

Many other important factors have been identified that may account for significant variations in biliary cholesterol secretion in the general population.[47] These factors may also have a genetic basis, but at present it is difficult to determine at what point—e.g., absorption, synthesis, conversion to bile salts — they may exert their influence on cholesterol metabolism. Some of the factors found to increase hepatic synthesis of cholesterol include hyperthyroidism, a biliary fistula or cholestyramine administration, and the ileal bypass procedure. Factors that may cause decreased hepatic cholesterol synthesis include cholesterol or chenodeoxycholic acid feeding, prolonged fasting, hypothyroidism, clofibrate, and estrogens. It is beyond the scope of this review to consider all these factors individually. Cholesterol–bile salt interactions occur in all the above situations and contribute to the net relative concentrations of cholesterol and bile salts in bile and to their respective pool sizes. Gradually we are beginning to recognize that, given the genetic, metabolic, and environmental conditions operative in a particular individual or homogeneous group, one can plot a spectrum of bile lithogenicity, i.e., shorter or longer times of day, or periods of time when cholesterol is supersaturated in bile and, if other forces are operative, is liable to nucleate crystals and begin the precipitation of stones.

ROLE OF THE GALLBLADDER

Local events occurring within the gallbladder may contribute to the hepatic secretion of lithogenic bile and certainly are accountable for precipitation of lithogenic bile within it. Just which events and their relative effects on the physical state of bile are questions which are still unsettled. The role of the gallbladder may be examined by asking the questions: What is the effect of cholecystectomy on stone formation and bile composition; and how do the functions of an intact gallbladder influence stone formation and bile composition?

Effect of Cholecystectomy

Abundant clinical reports attest to the efficacy of cholecystectomy in arresting spontaneous gallstone formation in humans. As early cholecystectomy is performed in younger and younger people, the incidence of secondary changes in the biliary tract, as well as of primary and recurrent common duct stones, is reduced.[48,49] In experimental animals, Van der Linden, Christensen, and Dam have demonstrated that cholecystectomy prevents the dietary induction of cholesterol gallstones in hamsters.[50] In human beings one cannot anticipate reports on the effects of prophylactic cholecystectomy among those who are unusually prone to stone formation, such as young Pima Indian women or children with thalassemia.

There have been many recent conflicting reports on the effect of cholecystectomy on hepatic bile composition.[41-46] In the relatively early reports of Shaffer[41] and Simmons[44] cholesterol-saturated bile became unsaturated following cholecystectomy. This change, which we have also noted in baboons following cholecystectomy,[51] would seem compatible with sequestration of part of the bile salt pool preoperatively and its redistribution throughout the enterohepatic circulation postcholecystectomy. Subsequently, the independent studies of Almond[43] and Pomare[42] failed to detect the same reversion of bile to a cholesterol-unsaturated state after cholecystectomy. Moreover, they noted either no change or a slight, further decrease in bile salt pool sizes, which had not been measured but would not have been expected in earlier studies. At about the same time yet another study[46] of bile in cholecystectomized patients demonstrated that secondary bile acids, particularly deoxycholic acid, had replaced cholic and chenodeoxycholic acid as the predominant bile acid component. Only one of the previous studies had also noted this;[42] whereas the cholate pool had dropped significantly in both studies, the chenodeoxycholate pool had slightly increased in one,[46] and decreased in the other.[42] Finally, in a study of cholecystectomized Southwest American Indians, Metzger and Grundy[45] demonstrated that there was no change from preoperative values for the hepatic secretion rates of bile acids, phospholipids, and cholesterol. Since these Indians had an elevated biliary cholesterol secretion preoperatively, they continued to secrete cholesterol-saturated lithogenic bile postoperatively. Finally, there was no tendency for an increased proportion of deoxycholic acid in bile after cholecystectomy. As one progresses through each study, it becomes increasingly hard to assimilate them all. Explanations that satisfy several studies' findings are inconsistent with at least one of the others. Although methodologic variations are apparent in the studies, these do not explain all the differences. It seems likely that differences in the patient populations studied and individual variations in enterohepatic metabolism will ultimately be clarified and account for our present confusion. At present, there appears to be strong suggestive evidence that the gallbladder, at least in some patients, exerts major feedback control on hepatic bile composition. It remains to be determined whether the radiographically functioning gallbladder has not already ceased to function in significant but inapparent ways, and that this may account for a lack of change in bile composition after cholecystectomy. On the other hand, Almond's and Metzger's reports serve to emphasize that the presence of lithogenic bile alone cannot account for its precipitation within the gallbladder, and that the salutary effect of cholecystectomy in deterring recurrent cholesterol stone formation may be, in some and possibly all instances, completely unrelated to any effects on biliary lipid composition or bile salt pool size.

Gallbladder Functions

The functions of the intact gallbladder are related to its capacity for mucous membrane transport, storage of bile, and muscular contraction. It is becoming apparent that physiologic, metabolic, and degenerative changes in gallbladder functions may alter the chemical composition and physical state of bile in a way that may contribute to precipitation of cholesterol and its retention and aggregation within the gallbladder. Selected aspects of these functions can be considered here.

Gross failure of the concentrating function of the gallbladder is frequently seen in advanced calculous disease of all types. Little is presently known about transient or selective or early malfunction of its mucous membrane. Ordinarily, the gallbladder membrane is impermeable to conjugated bilirubin, bile salts, lecithin, and cholesterol and concentrates them isosmotically with serum by a remarkable absorption of water and electrolytes.[52] Wheeler has reviewed the extensive physiologic data derived from animal studies[53] concerning the factors regulating active and passive transport processes across the gallbladder membrane. Evidence is accumulating which suggests that normal mucosal impermeability to biliary lipids may alter for metabolic analogues of bile acids and bilirubin, lecithin, and cholesterol derivatives. Membrane permeability properties have also been reported to change with overdistention of the gallbladder,[54] while proliferative change in the membrane epithelium has been reported in an instance of experimentally induced cholelithiasis.[55] Concentration of bile varies throughout the gallbladder, especially the solute concentration of cholesterol in the region of the gallbladder wall where crystal precipitation appears to originate.[56] A related aspect of membrane transport — mucous secretion into bile — appears important in the nucleation and growth of cholesterol crystals.[57,58] The viscosity of mucus and its tendency to form a gel and entrap crystals increase as the gallbladder membrane absorbs water and concentrates bile.[56,57] The amount of mucous membrane secretion, as elsewhere in the body, increases as a result of local irritation, which in turn might result from determinants of pH at the bile-mucosa interface; from dietary, drug, or endogenous metabolites in bile; and, of course, from solid stones.[57] In experimental diet- and drug-induced cholelithiasis in animals, increased mucous production often precedes stone formation,[52] and in human cholelithiasis both the nidus and the matrix of gallstones frequently are composed of mucopolysaccharides.[52]

Storage of bile in the gallbladder affects its own composition and that of the hepatic bile secreted into it. Storage capacity is related to the combined processes of concentration of bile and distention of the gallbladder to accommodate a larger volume. Together these processes enable the gallbladder to sequester over 95 per cent of the bile salt pool during a relatively short period of time, such as an overnight fast when no stimulus to emptying occurs. In addition to the ways in which variable membrane transport may alter gallbladder bile composition, other processes within the gallbladder can act on limpid bile. Accumulation of unconjugated bilirubin pigment or desquamated epithelial cells provides an excellent nidus for deposition of cholesterol.[52] Contamination by bacteria or pancreatic juices can lead to deconjugation of bile salts or hydrolysis of lecithin to lysolecithin, monoglycerides, and fatty acids, which effectively increase cholesterol saturation in gallbladder bile.[59] Concentration of bile can increase its solid weight content up to ten times; since both dilute and concentrated bile are continuously mixing in the gallbladder, stratification or layering of bile of different densities occurs. This and other physiochemical changes in bile relating to flow rates, fluid mechanics, micellar solubility, and time-dependent rate processes are being studied by Cussler and Evans,[56,60,61] Holzbach,[62] Carey,[63] and Higuchi[64] and appear to be crucial in setting the conditions for a change in the physical state of bile that is conducive to nucleation of cholesterol crystals, their net aggregation and growth, or their dissolution or dispersion.

The effect of storage of gallbladder bile on hepatic bile composition has been intensively studied by Thureborn[65] in humans, by Small[66] in rhesus monkeys, and by McSherry[11] in baboons. It is clear, as mentioned earlier, that the periodic sequestration of bile in the gallbladder, such as during an overnight fast or between meals, produces a temporary but acute decrease in rate of bile flow and a physiologic depletion of the circulating bile salt pool which results in production of cholesterol-saturated hepatic bile. Restoration of hepatic bile flow rate and chemical composition to a state more conducive to solubilizing cholesterol then partly depends on the degree and frequency of gallbladder contractile emptying.

The contractile function of the gallbladder, from the viewpoint of gallstone pathogenesis, is still of undetermined importance. Both concentrative and contractile functions are frequently impaired or lost in cases of long-standing chronic cholecystitis and cholelithiasis. Unfortunately, it is difficult to determine whether these changes are causative in or result from gallstone formation, or both. Similarly, concentrative and contractile functions are extremely difficult to study quantitatively in the human subject, in whom there may be a very indistinct dividing line between variations in normal function and early malfunction. At present, many suggestive correlations exist between cholelithiasis and stasis or impaired emptying of the gallbladder. These include changes in muscular tone or contractile ability in relation to pregnancy or female hormones;[67] vagotomy[68] or other conditions altering intestinal motility and cholecystokinin release; obstruction to emptying;[69] and increased extrahepatic biliary ductal pressure.[70] Clinical and experimental interest in these areas is rising and should result in further clarification of the role of the gallbladder in stone formation.

GENETIC, ENVIRONMENTAL, AND METABOLIC FACTORS

Genetic Factors

Genetic factors are probably involved in many of the pathogenic mechanisms leading to gallstones. This is suggested in human studies by the high incidence of cholesterol stones in diseases with an established genetic deficit, such as prebetahyperlipoproteinemia,[25] or by the comparative incidence of gallstones in diverse countries, such as Japan, Sweden, Finland, and the United States,[1] or in racially distinct populations, such as the Pima Indians of the Southwest United States[71] and the Masai natives of North Africa.[19] Further suggestive evidence is the marked difference in biliary lipid composition,[1] bile salt pool size,[5] and cholesterol secretion rates[16] in groups having a high incidence of stones. With regard to animal studies, many species, especially the nonhuman primates, have marked differences in their cholesterol and bile metabolism,[72,73] as evidenced by their proclivity to develop spontaneous[74,75] or diet-induced cholesterol gallstones[76] or hyperlipidemia.[77-78] Even within the same species of squirrel monkey, there appear to be different genotypes with marked variations in cholesterol metabolic pathways in response to cholesterol feeding.[78] However, at this time, no more than suggestive evidence has been mounted for genetic factors. Until more concrete evidence is forwarded, the remarkable individual variation in cholesterol metabolic pathways, which has also been found in the human, will only make differentiation of supposed genetic factors from environmental, degenerative, or other subtle factors difficult at this time.

Diet

Diet is emerging as a major determinant of bile composition and ultimately of potential to develop gallstones. Dietary manipulation has long been the main tool for inducing calculi in experimental animals.[9] Striking dietary differences between countries and racial populations having a very high or very low incidence of cholelithiasis and atherosclerosis present a strong alternate explanation of genetic theories.[79-81] Moreover, changes in a given racial population's type or incidence[81] of gallstones or both have been well correlated with changes in diet in that country or after migration to another country.[82] Very recently, two significant articles have been published correlating a cholesterol-lowering diet with increased incidence of gallstones[83] and a weight-reducing diet in obese subjects with marked change in bile composition to a cholesterol-saturated state.[84]

The mechanisms by which these diets may work are as varied as the diets themselves and include change in bile salt pool size,[76] increase in cholesterol concentration in bile,[34, 84] reduced dehydroxylation of bile salts,[85] and change in rate of gallbladder emptying and enterohepatic cycling of the bile salt pool.[85] This last mechanism may be of particular significance in light of the recent findings presented above that prolonged fasting results in gallbladder stasis and lithogenic hepatic bile, whereas increased gallbladder emptying and enterohepatic cycling of bile may render bile less saturated with cholesterol. Put another way, the frequency of eating may be as critical a determinant of bile composition as the bulk, caloric value, and chemical composition of the food ingested.

Drugs (Hormones, Bile Salts, Phenobarbital, Hypolipidemic Agents)

The liver and kidney are the major sites of endogenous and exogenous drug metabolism and excretion. Thus, it is not surprising that so many drugs, when investigated, are found to influence hepatic bile composition. From the viewpoint of gallstone pathogenesis, the drugs discussed below will be considered on the basis of their effect on cholesterol solubility in bile. As will be discussed later with lecithin feeding, or in the case of heparin, it is possible that many drugs may affect gallstone formation or dissolution by altering the physical rather than the chemical properties of bile. To be considered here are endogenous and pharmacologic levels of naturally occurring hormones and bile salts, as well as the sedative phenobarbital and hypolipidemic agents.

Estrogens represent one of many naturally occurring hormones that may exert profound effects on hepatobiliary tract function. For many years, female sex hormones have been implicated in bile stasis and delayed emptying of the gallbladder during the latter part of pregnancy or the menstrual cycle.[49,67] Many of these effects were presumably mediated through a generalized effect of estrogens on smooth muscle. However, it is increasingly obvious that estrogens, which are predominantly metabolized by the liver, have many primary effects on hepatic parenchymal cell function.[86] Lynn and Williams have reported decreased bile salt secretion relative to cholesterol in cholecystectomized rhesus monkeys administered estriol.[87] Deitrick and McSherry[88] noted decreased chenodeoxycholic acid pool size and synthesis in pregnant baboons. Pertsemlidis and Panveliwalla have shown increased hepatic cholesterol secretion in several cholecystectomized women following administration of oral contraceptives.[35]

These and other studies of the sex hormones should clarify the long disputed relationship of increased risk of cholelithiasis to pregnancy and, more recently, to oral contraceptives.[89] Many other hormones, particularly thyroid, cholecystokinin, and the other gastrointestinal hormones, significantly affect hepatobiliary tract function, but clear associations with human stone formation have yet to be established.

Although pharmacologic doses of bile salts have been used for years in the treatment of bile stasis, constipation, malabsorption, and other intestinal conditions, little was known about their metabolic effects until the last four years with the development of chenodeoxycholic acid therapy for dissolution of gallstones. The initial rationale for bile salt feeding derived from the studies of Small, Vlahcevic, Swell, Bell, and coworkers,[3, 5, 15, 90] who showed that many patients with gallstones have decreased cholate and chenodeoxycholate bile salt pool size, and that oral administration of bile salts markedly increases biliary phospholipid secretion relative to cholesterol, resulting in increased cholesterol solubility of bile. Subsequent studies by Danziger, Hofmann, Schoenfield and Thistle, and Bell demonstrated that chenodeoxycholic acid significantly expands the bile salt pool,[22,91] increases the solubility of cholesterol in bile,[92,93] and dissolves approximately 50 per cent of radiolucent gallstones.[91-93] Now it is becoming apparent that cholic acid, while it is effective in expanding the pools of cholic and deoxycholic acid, does so at the expense of a further reduction in chenodeoxycholic pool size and does not increase cholesterol solubility in bile or dissolve gallstones.[94] These factors and the finding that chenodeoxycholic acid lowers serum triglycerides significantly have raised the possibility that chenodeoxycholic acid is exerting profound effects at points in cholesterol and phospholipid metabolism, possibly in their synthetic pathways, and that these changes rather than expansion of the chenodeoxycholate pool account for its effectiveness in dissolving stones.[31, 37]

Phenobarbital also shows promise as a gallstone-dissolving agent. In addition to its value as a sedative, it is now well known as a potent inducer of hepatic microsomal enzyme activity[95] and has been used therapeutically to stimulate bile flow and bilirubin and bile salt transport in neonatal hyperbilirubinemic and cholestatic syndromes.[95] With regard to its effect on the lithogenicity of bile in lower animals, phenobarbital increases the activity of a 7α-hydroxylase, the rate-limiting enzyme step in the synthesis of bile acids from cholesterol and also increases hepatic phospholipid content and synthesis. Redinger and Small[96] have extended studies to nonhuman primates and shown that phenobarbital increases the solubility of bile for cholesterol by increasing bile salt synthesis, excretion, and pool size, as well as phospholipid secretion, without increasing cholesterol secretion. More recently, studies by Redinger[97] and Schoenfield[98] report a similar favorable effect of phenobarbital, alone or in combination with chenodeoxycholic acid, in patients with gallstones.

Drugs currently used in the treatment of hypolipidemia and atherosclerosis, e.g., cholestyramine, clofibrate, nicotinic acid, and D-thyroxine, emphasize the complex relationships between cholesterol and bile salt metabolism and, very likely, between these pathologic processes and cholesterol cholelithiasis. Levy[99] and Miettinen[100] have contributed recent comprehensive reviews on these agents. Both cholestyramine and thyroxine have long been used in the experimental production or prevention of gallstones.[9] Clofibrate causes a marked increase in cholesterol output in bile while decreasing cholesterol conversion to bile acids;[101] along with an increased lithogenicity of hepatic bile in patients on clofibrate, Grundy has reported instances of cholelithiasis.[33] It has already been noted, in the section on phospholipids, that both lecithin and chenodeoxycholic acid appear to have a serum triglyceride–lowering effect of therapeutic significance.

Acquired Metabolic Defects

In addition to genetic and environmental factors which may alter bile composition in favor of precipitation of cholesterol, there are acquired states of health or disease that are also associated with lithogenic bile and a higher incidence of cholelithiasis. We have already mentioned pregnancy, obesity, and the weight-losing state in association with prolonged dieting or the ileal bypass procedure. Diseases affecting bile salt metabolism, such as regional enteritis[102,103] and cirrhosis,[104] also have a high incidence of gallstones. It is beyond the scope of this review to go into the complex pathophysiology of these diseases. It is of interest, however, that a markedly decreased bile salt pool, as in the cirrhotic patient, need not lead to cholesterol stones, but here is associated with pigmented stones. The reason for this appears to be that the cirrhotic process results in markedly decreased phospholipid and cholesterol secretion in bile as well, and the bile remains unsaturated with respect to cholesterol.[104] Many other gaps in our knowledge of gallstone genesis and development still remain, and these gaps limit the success of our current attempts to reverse the process and dissolve gallstones.

GALLSTONE DISSOLUTION

Medical therapy to dissolve gallstones is still in an early, experimental stage. As such, it cannot be fairly compared at this time with the efficiency, specificity, and relative safety of cholecystectomy and common duct exploration. Nor is it yet clear which patients might be better treated by medical rather than surgical therapy, were both equally available. The purpose of this section, therefore, is to give a status report of efforts to dissolve gallstones, especially as they relate to current theories of cholesterol solubility in bile and stone formation.

At present there are two therapeutic possibilities for the nonsurgical treatment of cholelithiasis arising from defective bile salt or phospholipid secretion in bile: bile salt feeding and lecithin feeding. Stones in the gallbladder have decreased in size or dissolved following pharmacologic doses of oral chenodeoxycholic acid. Thistle and Hofmann[93] recently reported the current Mayo Clinic experience, in which partial or complete gallstone dissolution occurred in at least one-half of 53 patients treated for periods from six months to three years. The experience of others is comparable thus far.[92] The rationale for oral chenodeoxycholic acid therapy has been presented earlier. It now appears that chenodeoxycholic acid only dissolves about 50 per cent of radiolucent stones; that susceptible stones dissolve very slowly; and that cessation of therapy may result in reversion to lithogenic bile and reformation of stones in some individuals.[105] These observations raise questions about other factors controlling stone formation and suggest that a metabolic or genetic abnormality will maintain the stone-forming diathesis unless medical therapy is prolonged indefinitely or the gallbladder is removed. Many groups are studying these questions and the possible toxic or metabolic consequences of prolonged medical therapy.

Many of the patients with decreased bile salt pools who respond to chenodeoxycholic acid feeding also have decreased phospholipid secretion in bile.[25,30] This observation, as well as evidence that patients with gallstones may have significant defects in phospholipid metabolism, led Tompkins to try lecithin feeding.[32] This has increased phospholipid concentration in bile and been associated with a disappearance of cholesterol crystals, if not of gallstones, in some patients; moreover, as noted earlier, it has reversed the hypercholesterolemia and hypertriglyceridemia of other patients with serum lipoprotein disorders.[32] Although lecithin has not been as successful as chenodeoxycholic acid in dissolving gallstones, the reasons for this are emerging and may be surmounted. Higuchi[64] and Tao[61] have shown in vitro that, despite lecithin's great solubilizing capacity for cholesterol, once cholesterol stones have formed, other surface active forces predominate in bringing about their dissolution. In this latter respect, lecithin appears to act as a strong interfacial barrier to stone dissolution. However, there is hope that quaternary amines or other agents which overcome these interfacial barriers may render lecithin feeding as effective as bile salt feeding for the dissolution of gallstones.[106] Also, lecithin feeding, if it proves safer on a long-term basis than chenodeoxycholic acid feeding, could have a role in preventing gallbladder stone formation, or reformation once dissolved by bile salts, in patients at high risk to develop them.

Retained stones in the common bile duct have disappeared within two weeks following perfusion of the common duct with solutions of sodium cholate or heparin. In 1972, Way, Admirand, and Dunphy[107] reported 12 successful sodium cholate perfusions in 22 patients. In 1973, Lansford[108] reported success in five of six patients similarly treated. A possible scientific basis for the effectiveness of cholate was provided by the earlier studies of Small[109] and Earnest and Admirand,[110] who showed that bile salt solutions in vitro dissolve cholesterol from and decrease the size of cholesterol stones. Although it appears that mechanical flushing of the common duct does not account for the disappearance of retained stones,[107] the precise way in which cholate works is not clear. Way[111] and Lahana[106] have reached different conclusions about the relative effectiveness of cholate versus other bile salts for dissolving gallstones in vitro. Both Higuchi[64] and Evans and Cussler[60] have demonstrated multiple physiochemical factors that influence the rate and manner of dissolution of cholesterol stones. This is well illustrated by Gardner's[112] use of heparin to break up common duct stones. He has presented convincing evidence that the high ionic electronegativity of heparin disperses bile salt–lecithin micelles in bile, resulting in fragmentation of stones. To date, he has reported successful disappearance of retained stones in 21 out of 27 patients.[113] As might be expected, if different mechanisms of action are involved, heparin and sodium cholate together in vitro show even greater dissolution potential.[106] Others have not been successful with heparin perfusion in vivo or in vitro.[114] The ultimate clinical worth of all common duct perfusion agents will be determined only after more widespread trials.

It is not surprising that all gallbladder and common duct stones do not dissolve. The agents used are not universal solvents, and one cannot tell the chemical composition of a stone from the prevailing gallbladder or hepatic bile composition at the time of attempted dissolution. The composition of stones varies considerably from patient to patient. Even in the same patient, a single stone may have sequential layers of different crystalline compounds on its outer surface, reflecting a changing composition of bile and changing factors in stone growth during its development.[115] Reversing the forces that once caused precipitation of cholesterol crystals may no longer be possible years later in a malfunctioning biliary tract and, even then, may not be adequate to break down a calcified stone.

Despite the present limited success at gallstone dissolution, these efforts should be continued by those clinical and experimental investigators knowledgeable in the field. At present, each careful trial at gallstone dissolution advances our knowledge of gallstone formation. In the future, improved medical therapy may be an adjunct to the surgeon dealing with common duct stones and occasionally be a preferable initial treatment for gallbladder stones.

REFERENCES

1. Redinger, R. N., and Small, D. M.: Bile composition, bile salt metabolism and gallstones. Arch. Intern. Med. *130*:618, 1972.
2. Bourges, M., Small, D. M., and Dervichian, D. G.: Biophysics of lipidic associations. III. The quaternary system lecithin-bile-salt-cholesterol-water. Biochim. Biophys. Acta *144*:189, 1967.
3. Admirand, W. H., and Small, D. M.: The physiochemical basis of cholesterol gallstone formation in man. J. Clin. Invest. *47*:1043, 1968.
4. Thistle, J. L., and Schoenfield, L. J.: Lithogenic bile among young Indian women; lithogenic potential decreased with chenodeoxycholic acid. New Engl. J. Med. *284*:177, 1971.
5. Vlahcevic, Z. R., Bell, C. C., Jr., Gregory, D. H., Buker, G., Juttijudata, P., and Swell, L.: Relationship of bile acid pool size to the formation of lithogenic bile in female Indians of the Southwest. Gastroenterology *62*:73, 1972.
6. Dam, H., Kruse, I., Prange, I., Kallehauge, H. E., Fenger, H. J., and Krogh Jensen, M.: Studies on human bile. III. Composition of duodenal bile from surgical patients with and without uncomplicated gallstone disease. Z. Ernaehrungswiss. *10*:160, 1971.
7. Holzbach, R. T., Marsh, M., Olszewski, M., and Holam, K.: Cholesterol solubility in bile. Evidence that supersaturated bile is frequent in healthy man. J. Clin. Invest. *52*:1467, 1973.
8. Bell, C. C., Jr., McCormick, W. C., III, Gregory, D. H., et al.: Relationship of bile acid pool size to the formation of lithogenous bile in male Indians of the Southwest. Surg. Gynecol. Obstet. *134*:473, 1972.
9. Dam, H.: Determinants of cholesterol cholelithiasis in man and animals. Am. J. Med. *51*:596, 1971.
10. Metzger, A. L., Adler, R., Heymsfield, S., et al.: Diurnal-variation in biliary lipid composition. New Engl. J. Med. *288*:333, 1973.
11. McSherry, C. K., Glenn, F., and Javitt, N. B.: Composition of basal and stimulated hepatic bile in baboons, and the formation of cholesterol gallstones. Proc. Natl. Acad. Sci. USA *68*:1564, 1971.
12. Mufson, D., and Meksuwan, K.: Cholesterol solubility in lecithin bile salt systems. Science *177*:701, 1972.

13. Metzger, A. L., Heymsfield, S., and Grundy, S. M.: The lithogenic index—a numerical expression for the relative lithogenicity of bile. Gastroenterology 62:499, 1972.
14. Swell, L., Bell, C. C., Jr., Gregory, D. H., and Vlahcevic, Z. R.: The cholesterol saturation index of human bile. Dig. Dis. 19:261, 1974.
15. Vlahcevic, Z. R., Bell, C. C., Jr., and Swell, L.: Significance of the liver in the production of lithogenic bile in man. Gastroenterology 59:62, 1970.
16. Grundy, S. M., Metzger, A. L., and Adler, R.: Mechanisms of lithogenic bile formation in American Indian women with cholesterol gallstones. J. Clin. Invest. 51:3026, 1972.
17. Small, D. M., and Rapo, S.: Sources of abnormal bile in patients with cholesterol gallstones. New Engl. J. Med. 283:53, 1970.
18. Vlahcevic, Z. R., Bell, C. C., Jr., Buhac, I., Farrar, J. T., and Swell, L.: Diminished bile acid pool size in patients with gallstones. Gastroenterology 59:165, 1970.
19. Biss, K., Ho, K. J., Mikkelson, B., et al.: Some unique biologic characteristics of the Masai of East Africa. New Engl. J. Med. 284:694, 1971.
20. Javitt, N. B., and McSherry, C. K.: Pathogenesis of cholesterol gallstones. Hospital Practice 8:39, 1973.
21. Einarrson, K., and Hellstrom, K. J.: The formation of bile acids in patients with three types of hyperlipoproteinemia. Eur. J. Clin. Invest. 2:225, 1972.
22. Danziger, R. G., Hofmann, A. F., Schoenfield, J. J., and Thistle, J. L.: Dissolution of cholesterol gallstones by chenodeoxycholic acid. New Engl. J. Med. 286:1, 1972.
23. Swell, L., Entenman, C. M., Leong, G. F., and Holloway, R. J.: Bile acids and lipid metabolism. IV. Influence of bile acids on biliary and liver organelle phospholipids and cholesterol. Am. J. Physiol. 215:1390, 1968.
24. Tompkins, R. K., and King, W., III: Investigations of the enterobiliary metabolism of lecithin. Surgery 75:243, 1974.
25. Schersten, T.: Formation of lithogenic bile in man. Digestion 9:540, 1973.
26. Isaksson, B.: On the dissolving power of lecithin and bile salts for cholesterol in human bladder bile. Acta Soc. Med. Upsalien. 59:296, 1954.
27. Tompkins, R. K., Burke, L. G., Zollinger, R. M., and Cornwell, D. G.: The relationship of biliary phospholipid and cholesterol concentrations to the occurrence and dissolution of human gallstones. Ann. Surg. 172:936, 1970.
28. Nilsson, S., and Schersten, T.: Importance of bile acids for phospholipid secretion into human hepatic bile. Gastroenterology 57:525, 1969.
29. Nilsson, S., and Schersten, T.: Influence of bile acids on the synthesis of biliary phospholipids in man. Eur. J. Clin. Invest. 1:109, 1970.
30. Swell, L., Bell, C. C. Jr., and Vlahcevic, Z. R.: Relationship of bile acid pool size to biliary lipid excretion and the formation of lithogenic bile in man. Gastroenterology 61:716, 1971.
31. Bell, G. D., Lewis, B., Petrie, A., and Dowling, R. H.: Serum lipids in cholelithiasis; effect of chenodeoxycholic acid therapy. Br. Med. J. 3:520, 1973.
32. Tompkins, R. K., Corlin, R. F., Parkin, L. G., and King, W., III: Induced alterations in human serum lipids by prolonged phospholipid ingestion. Clin. Res. 21:276, 1973.
33. Grundy, S. M.: Cholesterol-bile acid interactions in gallstone pathogenesis. Hospital Practice 8:57, 1973.
34. Hofmann, A.: Can a cholesterol-lowering diet cause gallstones? New Engl. J. Med. 288:46, 1973.
35. Pertsemlidis, D., Panveliwalla, D., and Ahrens, E. J., Jr.: Effect of clofibrate and an estrogen-progesterone combination on fasting biliary lipids and cholic acid kinetics in men. Gastroenterology 66:565, 1974.
36. Small, D. M.: Prestone gallstone disease—is therapy safe? New Engl. J. Med. 284:214, 1971.
37. Hoffman, N. E., Hofmann, A. F., and Thistle, J. L.: Effect of bile acid feeding on cholesterol metabolism in gallstone patients. Mayo Clin. Proc. 49:236, 1974.
38. Grundy, S. M., and Metzger, A. L.: A physiologic method for estimation of hepatic secretion of biliary lipids in man. Gastroenterology 62:1200, 1972.

39. Grundy, S. M., Metzger, A. L., and Adler, R. D.: Mechanisms of lithogenic bile formation in American Indian women with cholesterol gallstones. J. Clin. Invest. *51*:3026, 1972.
40. Faloon, W. W.: Gallstone prophylaxis and therapy (report of a conference). Dig. Dis. *19*:81, 1974.
41. Shaffer, E. A., Braasch, J. W., and Small, D. M.: Bile composition at and after surgery in normal persons and patients with gallstones. New Engl. J. Med. *287*:1317, 1972.
42. Pomare, E. W., and Heaton, K. W.: The effect of cholecystectomy on bile salt metabolism. Gut *14*:753, 1973.
43. Almond, H. R., Vlahcevic, Z. R., Bell, C. C., Jr., Gregory, D. H., and Swell, L.: Bile acid pools, kinetics and biliary lipid composition before and after cholecystectomy. New Engl. J. Med. *289*:1213, 1973.
44. Simmons, F., Ross, A. P. J., and Bouchier, I. A. D.: Alterations in hepatic bile composition after cholecystectomy. Gastroenterology *63*:446, 1972.
45. Adler, R. D., Metzger, A. L., and Grundy, S. M.: Biliary lipid secretion before and after cholecystectomy in American Indians with cholesterol gallstones. Gastroenterology *66*:1212, 1974.
46. Hepner, G. W., Hofmann, A. F., Malagelada, J. R., Szczepanik, P. A., and Klein, P. B.: Increased bacterial degradation of bile acids in cholecystectomized patients. Gastroenterology *66*:556, 1974.
47. Bortz, W. M.: On the control of cholesterol synthesis. Metabolism *22*:1507, 1973.
48. Glenn, F.: Retained calculi within the biliary ductal system. Ann. Surg. *179*:528, 1974.
49. Morrissey, K., and Eisenmenger, W.: Medical aspects of diseases of the gallbladder and biliary tree. Am. J. Med. *51*:642, 1971.
50. Van der Linden, W., Christensen, F., and Dam, H: Cholecystectomy and gallstone formation in the golden hamster. Acta Chir. Scand. *118*:113, 1959.
51. McSherry, C. K., Morrissey, K., May, P., Javitt, N. B., and Glenn, F.: The role of hepatic bile production in gallstone formation in baboons. Ann. Surg. *178*:669, 1973.
52. Bouchier, I. A. D., and Freston, J. W.: The aetiology of gallstones. Lancet *1*:340, 1968.
53. Wheeler, H. O.: Concentrating function of the gallbladder. Am. J. Med. *51*:588, 1971.
54. Hall, R. C., Crosby, J. T., and Tepperman, J.: Bile flow and enlargement of the gallbladder in experimental cholelithiasis. Surg. Forum *22*:384, 1971.
55. Ely, J. W., Hall, R. C., and Tepperman, J.: Mucus production in gallstone formation — autoradiographs using tritiated galactose. Surg. Forum *22*:383, 1971.
56. Cussler, E. L., Evans, D. F., and DePalma, R. G.: A model for gallbladder function and cholesterol gallstone formation. Proc. Natl. Acad. Sci. USA *67*:400, 1970.
57. Hulten, O.: Formation of gallstones I. Acta Chir. Scand. *134*:125, 1968.
58. Womack, N. A., Zeppa, R., and Irvin, G. L.: The anatomy of gallstones. Ann. Surg. *157*:670, 1963.
59. Inoue, T., and Juniper, K., Jr.: The effect of sodium oleate on cholesterol solubility in bile salt-lecithin model systems. Dig. Dis. *18*:1067, 1973.
60. Evans, D. F., and Cussler, E. L.: Physico-chemical considerations in gallstone pathogenesis. Hospital Practice *9*:133, 1974.
61. Tao, J. C., Cussler, E. L., and Evans, D. F.: Accelerating gallstone dissolution. Proc. Natl. Acad. Sci. USA *71*:3917, 1974.
62. Holzbach, R. T., and Pak, C. Y. C.: Metastable supersaturation-physicochemical studies provide new insights into formation of renal and biliary tract stones. Am. J. Med. *56*:141, 1974.
63. Carey, M. C., and Small, D. M.: Micelle formation by bile salts. Arch. Intern Med. *130*:506, 1972.
64. Higuchi, W. I., Sjuib, F., Mufson, D., Simonelli, A. P., and Hofmann, A. F.: Dissolution kinetics of gallstones: physical model approach. J. Pharm. Sci. *63*(6):942, 1973.
65. Thureborn, E.: Human hepatic bile: Composition changes due to altered enterohepatic circulation. Acta Chir. Scand. Suppl. 303, 1962.

66. Dowling, R. H., Mack, E., and Small, D. M.: Primate biliary physiology. IV. Biliary lipid secretion and bile composition after acute and chronic interruption of the enterohepatic circulation in the rhesus monkey. J. Clin. Invest. 50:1917, 1971.

67. Nilsson, S., and Stattin, S.: Gallbladder emptying during the normal menstrual cycle. Acta Chir. Scand. 133:648, 1967.

68. Mujahed, Z., and Evans, J. A.: The relationship of cholelithiasis to vagotomy. Surg. Gynecol. Obstet. 133:656, 1971.

69. Gilsdorf, R. B.: The effect of simulated gallstones on gallbladder pressure and bile flow response to eating. Surg. Gynecol. Obstet. 138:161, 1974.

70. Strasberg, S. M., Dorn, B. C., Small, D. M., and Egdahl, R. H.: The effect of biliary tract pressure on bile flow, bile salt secretion, and bile salt synthesis in the primate. Surgery 70:140, 1971.

71. Comess, L. J., Bennett, P. H., and Burch, T. A.: Clinical gallbladder disease in Pima Indians: its high prevalence in contrast to Framingham, Massachusetts. New Engl. J. Med. 277:894, 1967.

72. Eggen, D. A.: Cholesterol metabolism in Rhesus monkey, squirrel monkey, and baboon. J. Lipid Res. 15:139, 1974.

73. Schoenfield, L. J.: Animal models of gallstone formation. Gastroenterology 63:189, 1972.

74. Martin, D. E., Wolf, R. C., and Houser, W. D.: Naturally occurring cholelithiasis in a rhesus monkey and its effects on plasma and biliary lipid concentrations. Am. J. Vet. Res. 34:971, 1973.

75. Glenn, F., and McSherry, C. K.: The baboon and experimental cholelithiasis. Arch. Surg. 100:105, 1970.

76. Osuga, T., and Portman, O. W.: Experimental formation of gallstones in the squirrel monkey. Proc. Soc. Exp. Biol. Med. 136:722, 1971.

77. Armstrong, M. L., Connor, W. E., and Warner, E. D.: Tissue cholesterol concentration in the hypercholesterolemic rhesus monkey. Arch. Pathol. 87:87, 1969.

78. Lofland, H. B., Jr., Clarkson, T. B., St. Clair, R. W., and Lehner, N. D. M.: Studies on the regulation of plasma cholesterol levels in squirrel monkeys of two genotypes. J. Lipid Res. 13:39, 1972.

79. Walker, A. R. P.: Some aspects of nutritional research in South Africa. Nutr. Rev. 14:321, 1956.

80. Nakayama, F., and Van der Linden, W.: Bile composition: Sweden vs. Japan. Am. J. Surg. 122:12, 1971.

81. Nakayama, F., and Miyake, H.: Changing state of gallstone disease in Japan. Composition of stones and treatment of the condition. Am. J. Surg. 120:794, 1970.

82. Malhotra, S. L.: Epidemiological study of cholelithiasis among railroad workers in India with special reference to causation. Gut 9:2920, 1968.

83. Sturdevant, R. A. L., Pearce, M. L., and Dayton, S.: Increased gallstone prevalence in men on serum cholesterol-lowering diets. New Engl. J. Med. 288:24, 1973.

84. Schreibman, P. H., Pertsemlidis, D., Liu, G. C. K., and Ahrens, E. H., Jr.: Lithogenic bile—a consequence of weight reduction. J. Clin. Invest. 53:72a, 1974.

85. Pomare, E. W., and Heaton, K. W.: Alteration of bile salt metabolism by dietary fibre (bran). Br. Med. J.4:262, 1973.

86. Inglefinger, F. J.: Estrogens and gallstones (editorial). New Engl. J. Med. 290:51, 1974.

87. Lynn, J., Williams, L. F., and O'Brien, J.: Effects of estrogen upon bile: Implications with respect to gallstone formation. Ann. Surg. 178:514, 1973.

88. Deitrick, J. W., McSherry, C. K., Javitt, N. B., and Glenn, F.: Bile salt kinetics in the pregnant baboon: a new model for the study of gallbladder function. Gastroenterology 65:536, 1973.

89. Boston Collaborative Drug Surveillance Program. Oral contraceptives and venous thromboembolic disease, surgically confirmed gallbladder disease, and breast tumors. Lancet 1:1399, 1973.

90. Bell, C. C., Jr., Vlahcevic, Z. R., and Swell, L: Alterations in the lipids of human

hepatic bile after the oral administration of bile salts. Surg. Gynecol. Obstet. *132*:36, 1971.

91. Thistle, J. L.: Cholesterol gallstone dissolution. Arch. Surg. *107*:831, 1973.
92. Bell, G. D., Whitney, B., and Dowling, R. H.: Gallstone dissolution in man using chenodeoxycholic acid. Lancet *2*:1213, 1972.
93. Thistle, J. L., and Hofmann, A. F.: Efficacy and specificity of chenodeoxycholic acid therapy for dissolving gallstones. New Engl. J. Med. *289*:655, 1973.
94. LaRusso, N. F., Hoffman, N. E., Hofmann, A. F., Northfield, T. C., and Thistle, J. L.: Differing effects of primary bile acid ingestion on biliary lipid secretion in gallstone patients. Why chenodeoxycholic acid dissolves gallstones. Gastroenterology *66*:729, 1974.
95. Sharp, H. L., and Mirkin, B. L.: Effect of phenobarbital on hyperbilirubinemia, bile acid metabolism, and microsomal enzyme activity in chronic intrahepatic cholestasis of childhood. Pediatrics *81*:116, 1972.
96. Redinger, R. N., and Small, D. M.: The effect of phenobarbital upon bile salt synthesis and pool size, biliary lipid secretion and bile composition. J. Clin. Invest. *52*:161, 1973.
97. Redinger, R. N.: The effect of phenobarbital on biliary lipid metabolism. Gastroenterology *66*:763, 1974.
98. Coyne, M. J., Bonorris, G. G., Goldstein, L. I., Lahana, D. A., and Schoenfield, L. J.: Dissolution of gallstones by chenodeoxycholic acid and phenobarbital. Gastroenterology *66*:679, 1974.
99. Levy, R., Morganroth, J., and Rifkind, B. M.: Drug therapy; treatment of hyperlipidemia. New Engl. J. Med. *290*:1295, 1974.
100. Miettinen, T. A.: Effect of drugs on bile acid and cholesterol excretion. Excerpta Medica (Lipid Metabolism and Atherosclerosis) #283:77, 1974.
101. Grundy, S. M.: Treatment of hypercholesterolemia by interference with bile acid metabolism. Arch. Intern. Med. *130*:638, 1972.
102. Heaton, K. W., and Read, A. E.: Gallstones in patients with disorders of the terminal ileum and disturbed bile salt metabolism. Br. Med. J. *3*:494, 1969.
103. Cohen, S., Kaplan, M., Gottleib, L., and Patterson, J.: Liver disease and gallstones in regional enteritis. Gastroenterology *60*:237, 1971.
104. Vlahcevic, Z. R., Yoshida, T., Juttijudata, P., Bell, C. C., Jr., and Swell, L.: Biliary lipid secretion in patients with cirrhosis and its relevance to gallstone formation. Gastroenterology *64*:298, 1973.
105. Thistle, J. L., Paulina, Y. S., Hofmann, A. F., and Ott, B. J.: Prompt return of bile to supersaturated state followed by gallstone recurrence after discontinuance of chenodeoxycholic acid therapy. Gastroenterology *66*:789, 1974.
106. Lahana, D. A., Bonorris, G. G., and Schoenfield, L. J.: Gallstone dissolution in vitro by bile acids, heparin and quaternary amines. Surg. Gynecol. Obstet. *138*:683, 1974.
107. Way, L. W., Admirand, W. H., and Dunphy, J. F.: Management of choledocholithiasis. Ann. Surg. *176*:347, 1972.
108. Lansford, C., and Kern, F.: The treatment of retained stones in the common bile duct with sodium cholate infusion. Gut *15*:48, 1974.
109. Small, D. M.: The formation of gallstones. Adv. Intern. Med. *16*:243, 1970.
110. Earnest, D. E., and Admirand, W. H.: The effects of individual bile salts in cholesterol solubilization and gallstone dissolution. Gastroenterology *60*:772, 1971.
111. Way, L. W.: *In vitro* dissolution of cholesterol gallstones. Surg. Forum *24*:412, 1973.
112. Gardner, B.: Experience with the use of intracholedochal heparinized saline for the treatment of retained common duct stones. Ann. Surg. *177*:240, 1973.
113. Gardner, B., Dennis, C., and Patti, J.: Heparin dissolution of gallstones: experimental and clinical observations. Presented at the Assoc. for Acad. Surg., Nov., 1973.
114. Romero, R., and Butterfield, W. C.: Heparin and gallstones. Am. J. Surg. *127*:687, 1974.
115. Sutor, D. J., and Wooley, S. E.: The sequential deposition of crystalline material in gallstones: Evidence for changing gallbladder bile composition during the growth of some stones. Gut *15*:130, 1974.

Chapter Four

CHOLELITHIASIS

INCIDENCE

The incidence or occurrence of cholelithiasis varies according to the race and origin of the population studied. Some peoples have an extremely high occurrence rate of cholelithiasis. Among those best known are the Indians of the southwestern United States, particularly the Pima Indians but in some degree the Chippaqua and Navaho Indians. Gallbladder x-ray studies of the Pima Indians, for instance, have revealed gallstones in 73 per cent of all women between the ages of 25 and 34.[5] The same study revealed the incidence of gallstones to be 48.6 per cent among 596 Indians studied. The group contained equal numbers of men and women.

Sweden seems to be another area where gallstones are very common. A recent study done from autopsy material there found that stones were present in 57 per cent of women and 32 per cent of men over the age of 20.[2] The incidence rose with advancing age.

The true incidence of cholelithiasis in the United States is not known; on the other hand, it is known to be very common, since over 300,000 cholecystectomies are performed in the United States every year, and the great majority of these are done for gallstones. In a ten-year study of men and women aged 30 to 60, 8 per cent of the men and women were found to have gallbladder disease.[1] Various autopsy series give different incidences of gallstones; for instance, one quotes incidences of 16.8 per cent in women and 7.8 per cent in men over age 20, but here also the incidence of gallstones seems to increase with age.[3]

In some countries the incidence of gallstones is apparently quite low. In Kampala, Uganda, surveys have shown that gallstones are present in only 1.35 per cent of subjects between the ages of 35 and 54;[2] these figures have been derived from autopsy examinations which also revealed that most of the stones were pure bilirubin stones. Studies of the composition of bile seem to indicate that the people with a high incidence of gallstones have bile that is saturated or supersaturated with cholesterol and may have a reduced bile acid pool. Conversely, in the areas of low incidence of gallstones, the bile of the population as a rule is undersaturated with cholesterol.[6,8]

There is also evidence for a different bile composition and thus probably a different etiology of gallstones in different civilizations. For instance, in the typical Western country the majority of gall-stones are found to be composed of cholesterol or a mixture of choles-terol with other components of bile, such as bilirubin and calcium. In the Far East in the past, the majority of gallstones were of the bile pigment variety, or mainly composed of bile pigment and bilirubin, whereas in later years investigations have shown a marked increase in cholesterol stones in this same population and a corresponding de-crease in the number of bile pigment stones. In areas where bile pigment stones prevail, the occurrence of gallstones in men and women is usually approximately equal and is evident at a younger age, whereas in areas where cholesterol stones predominate, the usual sex difference found in the West prevails — that is, three women with gallstones are usually found to every one man harboring the same disease, and the stones are more common with advanced age.

SYMPTOMS

Probably the most common complaint of patients suffering from cholelithiasis is some kind of dyspepsia. The dyspepsia of chole-lithiasis is very easily described as a bloated feeling after eating with increased gaseous eruptions and uncomfortable epigastric distress, occasionally leading to nausea and vomiting. The symptom of dyspep-sia is not specific to gallbladder disease, however, and is one of the symptoms that sometimes remains with the patient even after chole-cystectomy has been performed. Usually, though, up to half or some-times more than half of the patients whose complaint is dyspepsia are relieved following cholecystectomy. Biliary colic is of course the best known symptom of cholelithiasis; usually biliary colic comes from a stone being impacted or passing through the cystic duct. Biliary colic is of longer duration than intestinal colic and quite often presents a more steady and unremitting pain than is expected in colic. The pain is usually in the midepigastrium and quite commonly radiates to the back underneath the right shoulderblade. The radiation of pain in biliary colic can vary considerably, however. Radiation may be around the body in a girdle-type fashion, and when this symptom occurs, it probably is related to spasm of the ampulla of Vater or possibly to a stone located in that area. The pain often is referred to the upper right quadrant and to the midepigastrium or shifts from the epigastrium to the right upper quadrant, and occasionally patients complain more about back pain and true epigastric pain.

NATURAL HISTORY AND ITS INFLUENCE ON TREATMENT

At the moment surgery is the only accepted curative approach to gallstones. It is likely to remain so until methods of dissolving gallstones have reached a more predictable stage and the possible side effects of such treatment have been fully evaluated. Most physicians would agree that patients who have suffered some of the complications of gallstone disease or who are reasonably symptomatic should be advised to undergo surgery, should their health permit. There is still debate about what to do for or advise patients who are discovered to have gallstones and yet do not suffer significant symptoms. There is probably little disagreement that operations should not be advised for persons in precarious health until the need is clearly established by symptomatology. The debate revolves around what to advise the young or middle-aged person in good health when gallstones are accidentally discovered. It is well established that surgery for gallstones can be performed with the least mortality and morbidity when it is done on a young person on an elective basis. Morbidity and mortality rise steadily with advanced age of the patient and with the advancement of the disease process, the most serious complications being acute cholecystitis, common duct stones, biliary enteric fistulas, and carcinoma of the gallbladder. Most physicians are aware of the reasonably common finding of gallstones at autopsy, often in old people who have had minimal or few symptoms of the disease; thus they are loath to advise operation until it is clinically necessary. One reason for this unwillingness to urge surgery on a preventive basis has been the fact that few studies have been done on the fate of the patient with asymptomatic gallstones.

Two studies are now available on the fate of the patient with asymptomatic gallstones. In 1960 Lund[4] reported on 526 patients followed for from 5 to 20 years. In this period of time almost half of the patients developed symptoms, and three developed carcinoma of the gallbladder. In 1966 Weinkert[7] reported on 781 patients followed for more than 11 years. Of these patients 49 per cent were still free of symptoms and 33 per cent had developed serious complications; in this last group, three patients developed carcinoma of the gallbladder, and seven died from their disease. The author also reported on patients who underwent elective surgery for asymptomatic gallstones and on a second group of patients on whom surgery was performed soon after the first symptoms appeared. A much higher incidence of common duct exploration was found in the group of patients in whom surgery had been delayed following the diagnosis of gallstones.

It would therefore seem indicated to advise elective cholecystectomy for persons in good health who are found to have asymptomatic gallstones, since less than half are likely to be still free of symptoms ten years from discovery.

REFERENCES

1. Friedman, G. D., Kaund, W. B., and Dauber, T. R.: The epidemiology of gallbladder disease. J. Chronic Dis. *19*:273, 1966.
2. Heaton, K. W.: The epidemiology of gallstones and suggested etiology. Clinics in Gastroenterology 2:67, 1973.
3. Lieber, M. M.: The incidence of gallstones and their correlation with other disease. Ann. Surg. *135*:394, 1952.
4. Lund, J.: Surgical indications in cholelithiasis. Ann. Surg. *151*:153, 1960.
5. Sampliner, R. E., Bennett, P. H., Cornell, L. J., Rose, F. A., and Burch, T. A.: Gallbladder disease in Pima Indians. New Engl. J. Med. 283:1358, 1970.
6. Thistle, J. L., and Schoenfield, L. J.: Lithogenic bile among young Indian women; lithogenic potential decreased with chenodeoxycholic acid. New Engl. J. Med. *284*:177, 1971.
7. Weinkert, A., and Robertson, B.: Natural course of gallstone disease. Gastroenterology *50*:376, 1966.
8. Vlahcevic, Z. R., Bell, C. C., Jr., Gregory, D. H., Buker, G., Juttijudata, P., and Swell, L.: Relationship of bile acid pool size to the formation of lithogenic bile in female Indians of the Southwest. Gastroenterology *62*:73, 1972.

Chapter Five

INFLAMMATORY DISEASES OF THE BILIARY TRACT

ACUTE CHOLECYSTITIS

Etiology

About 20 per cent of people entering hospitals for surgery of the biliary tract do so because of acute cholecystitis. Usually the acute inflammation of the gallbladder is associated with stones. Approximately 90 to 95 per cent of patients with acute cholecystitis develop this complication because of calculi in the gallbladder.[9] The common cause of acute cholecystitis with stones is the impaction of a stone in the ampulla or cystic duct of the gallbladder. This impaction commonly results after a large meal, the gallbladder exerting maximum efforts to empty itself of bile following the stimulation of the meal. As a result a stone, usually of a reasonably small size, is impacted in the ampulla or cystic duct, causing the obstruction. Direct pressure of the stone on the mucosa of the gallbladder results in ischemia, necrosis, and ulceration. There is edema and swelling in the layers of the gallbladder wall. This swelling impedes the venous drainage of the organ, which in turn increases and extends the intensity of the inflammatory process, which may result in intramural bleeding and ultimately arterial ischemia with necrosis of the gallbladder wall, as well as perforation.[9]

Although mechanical obstruction of the cystic duct is the most common cause of acute cholecystitis and the most significant factor in its development, bacterial infection also plays a role. In the past bacterial infection was commonly the cause of acute cholecystitis

39

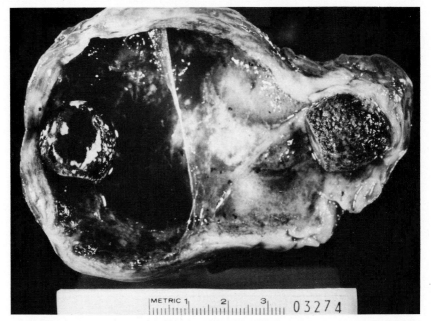

Figure 5-1 Acute cholecystitis. The gallbladder has greatly thickened walls with a necrotic mucosal lining. The impacted stone causing the acute attack is seen still in place in the ampulla of the gallbladder in the right end of the specimen.

in conditions such as typhoid fever. Today acute cholecystitis associated with typhoid fever is rarely encountered, but bacteria still play a major role in the progress of the disease. Bacterial cultures are obtained more often from gallbladders removed for acute cholecystitis than from those removed for chronic inflammation. Cultures have been obtained from up to 50 per cent of the gallbladders removed for acute or chronic cholecystitis, and the most common bacteria found were *E. coli, Klebsiella, Aerobacter,* enterococci, and staphylococci.[9] At times a bacterial infection may be the primary cause of acute cholecystitis, even though stones are usually present. Other proposed causes of acute cholecystitis are overconcentration of bile in the gallbladder, which results in damage to the mucosa of the organ, and the presence of large amounts of pancreatic ferments in the gallbladder bile.[10]

Acute cholecystitis is frequently seen in people with long-standing impairment of renal function and in those in whom the blood supply to the gallbladder is affected by arteritis or collagen disease, such as periarteritis nodosa or malignant hypertension. Acute cholecystitis occurs frequently in the immediate postoperative period of major operations.[8,17] Sometimes this occurs when the patient already has gallstones and is possibly related to the intake of food after prolonged periods of fasting, resulting in impaction of stones in the neck of the gallbladder similar to that occurring in attacks of ordinary acute cholecystitis. Other patients, however, develop acalculous cholecystitis following major surgery and major trauma.[11,12,14,15,16,21] The etiology of this acute acalculous cholecystitis is not clear, but several factors may be involved. A suggestion has been made that increased amounts of breakdown products of hemoglobin in the blood may injure the gallbladder mucosa, since this occurs in sepsis or after multiple massive transfusions. Dehydration, fever, and prolonged intravenous alimentation also predispose to overconcentration of bile in the gallbladder and thus damage the wall.

Emphysematous cholecystitis is a variety of acute cholecystitis[28] in which clostridia or other gas-forming organisms, usually *E. coli*, produce gas inside the biliary tract. The gas may be both intraluminal and intramural. Occasionally the wall of the gallbladder may weaken and allow gas to escape into the free peritoneal cavity, producing pneumoperitoneum with free air.[29] Emphysematous cholecystitis is found more often in men than in women, and it occurs frequently in

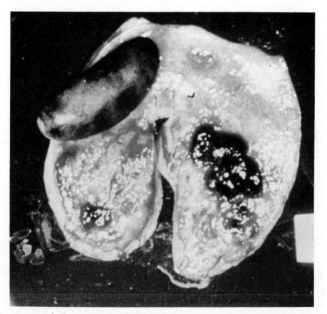

Figure 5–2 Acute cholecystitis with hemobilia. Acute cholecystitis is usually caused by the stones impacted in the ampulla of the gallbladder. The impaction of the stones causes swelling and edema, which first leads to venous congestion and later may interfere with the arterial blood supply to the gallbladder. This stone had eroded through the wall of the gallbladder into the cystic artery, which bled profusely into the gallbladder. The stone was dislodged and blood was passed through the cystic duct into the bile duct and the intestinal tract, and the patient developed melena.

diabetics.[30] Calculi are usually found in the gallbladder, but some reports indicate that only half of the patients have stones.[31] The diagnosis, similar to that of acute cholecystitis, is made by plain films showing intraluminal or intramural air in the gallbladder and sometimes in the bile duct. The treatment is the same as that for acute cholecystitis. Surgery should be performed as soon as the patient's condition permits. Preoperative preparation with antibiotics and supportive measures is very important, but when the patient is deteriorating, prompt drainage is essential.

Mortality is high in emphysematous cholecystitis, reflecting the poor condition of the patient.

Finally it should be mentioned that neoplasms of the gallbladder may cause acute cholecystitis, not only by obstructing the lumen of the gallbladder, as do stones, but also by invading and damaging the walls of the organ itself and thus predisposing to and encouraging infection. About 1 per cent of gallbladders removed when the diagnosis is acute cholecystitis are found to contain malignant tumors.[18]

Symptoms

In early stages the symptoms of patients with acute cholecystitis do not vary much from those of people with chronically inflamed gallbladders containing stones. There is onset of acute pain, usually epigastric in origin and perhaps referred more to the right side than to the left, although the pit of the stomach is the usual reference point. Along with this pain there is loss of appetite, a feeling of oppression, distention, and occasionally nausea. The pain frequently extends to the back underneath the right scapula. Initially the pain is often colicky, but as the inflammatory process increases, it becomes steady and boring, and tenderness is evident on palpation of the right upper quadrant. Uncommonly there are fever and chills at the onset of an attack of acute cholecystitis.

Physical Examination

Physical examination of the patient with acute cholecystitis in the early stages may reveal mild tenderness in the right upper quadrant with shock tenderness over the costal margin, and some minor guarding in the upper abdomen with some diminution in intestinal sounds on auscultation. A mass is usually not palpable in the early stages of acute cholecystitis, but in a large number of instances one does develop over the next 24 hours and is either the enlarged, tender gallbladder or the omentum and transverse colon wrapped around the inflamed organ. This mass usually moves with respiration and is not necessarily in the typical anatomic location of the gallbladder. Quite often it may present in the right flank, an area where a kidney is to be expected, and may indeed at times be palpable by bimanual examination.

Laboratory Findings

X-ray examination of the abdomen in the early stages of acute cholecystitis usually is not rewarding except as an aid in excluding other diseases. The gallstones usually are not visible on flat plates of the abdomen, but an estimated 10 per cent do show because of the calcium content and, when visible, will aid a great deal in arriving at the diagnosis. When acute cholecystitis has progressed and, as occasionally happens, a stone has eroded into the intestinal lumen, air can be seen in the biliary tree, aiding in the diagnosis of acute cholecystitis involving communication with the intestinal tract and the possibility of gallstone ileus. The temperature is usually only moderately elevated in the early stages but may rise rapidly and on occasion be septic in nature due to empyema or purulent infection within the gallbladder itself. The white blood count is elevated with a shift to the younger forms, and a white cell count of 14,000 to 20,000 is not unusual.

The differential diagnosis in acute cholecystitis usually involves perforated peptic ulcer, acute appendicitis, a primary inflammatory disease of the liver itself, and, rarely, rapid decompensation of the heart with engorgement of the liver and right lower lobe pneumonia. Pancreatitis is a common differential diagnostic problem, particularly because it may present without cholecystitis or may be part of the picture of acute cholecystitis itself.

There can be mild jaundice associated with uncomplicated acute cholecystitis, that is, without stones in the common duct. This jaundice, though, is usually mild; it is rarely over 2 to 3 mg and is caused by spread of the inflammation from the ampulla of the gallbladder over onto the common duct and by pressure from the ampulla of the gallbladder, which impacts itself in the foramen of Winslow and thus exerts pressure on the common duct. Usually at this time there is also mild elevation of the SGOT and SGPT, giving evidence of damage to the liver due to direct inflammatory spread from the gallbladder and to mild obstruction of the common duct. Although jaundice is frequently caused by inflammatory reaction or pressure from the ampulla of the gallbladder, it is more often derived from the common causes of obstruction, such as common duct stones. Among 1130 patients with acute cholecystitis operated upon at the New York

Hospital, common duct explorations were undertaken in 137 or 12 per cent of the group. Stones were found in the ducts of 59 per cent of those explored. This compares well with figures from the same institution, in which 14 per cent of patients with chronic cholecystitis underwent common duct exploration, and stones were removed from the duct in 64 per cent of those explored.[9] Corlette[5] estimates that jaundice is found in 17 to 30 per cent of patients with acute cholecystitis. He believes that most of these patients have an organic explanation for the jaundice, i.e., of 37 patients, 15 were found to have common duct stones, five had carcinoma, three had stricture, and eight were believed to have passed a stone. Of the 37 patients studied, only three were believed to have had no organic explanation for the jaundice, which might have been due to inflammatory reaction or pressure from the gallbladder ampulla. Watkin[20] found 32 jaundiced patients among 144 with acute cholecystitis; of those 32, 73 per cent had stones in the common bile duct, whereas only 6.5 per cent of the patients without jaundice had stones. Every patient with jaundice and acute cholecystitis must thus be suspected of common duct stone.

Timing of Operation

The surgery of acute cholecystitis is only rarely emergency surgery. More and more, though, the surgery is being performed during the acute attack rather than after the acute process has subsided, so that an elective cholecystectomy can be performed a few months later. One reason for the trend toward early operation in acute cholecystitis is the unpredictable course of the disease; that is, perforation may occur even while the patient is under observation in a hospital.[1,7] A second reason is that early operation shortens the hospital stay and time lost from work for the patient. A third reason is that a well-trained surgeon can perform a cholecystectomy safely during the acute attack, with a morbidity and mortality rate comparable to and better than that obtained from conservative treatment with delayed operations.[9-13]

In 1959 McCubbrey and Thieme analyzed the course of 345 patients with acute cholecystitis. All the patients were treated by nonsurgical methods except when needed. Of these patients, 191 were operated upon with a total mortality of 4.7 per cent. The authors point out that theirs is a community hospital without some of the amenities available in large teaching centers.[13] In 1961, a series of 1130 patients with acute cholecystitis treated surgically at the New York Hospital revealed a total mortality of 2.9 per cent, and in 1970 a series from Ohio[22] was published, consisting of 4206 patients who underwent cholecystectomy for acute cholecystitis, with a mortality of 3.5 per cent.

It should be remembered, though, that the mortality in surgery for acute cholecystitis often involves those patients who undergo only cholecystostomy.[9] McCubbrey and Thieme properly point out that the mortality in acute cholecystitis is influenced not only by the type of treatment applied but also by the type of patient. It is well accepted that the mortality and morbidity mainly involve the older patient, and the causes of death have changed markedly over the past decades. Infection and sepsis were determining factors in the results of surgery prior to 1950 but now take a back seat to cerebrovascular and cardiovascular complications, which prevail among the elderly. This does not imply that infection has been eliminated as a problem but rather that it can be better controlled by the availability of a steady flow of new and powerful antibiotics.[9] Infection[6] is still a major cause of morbidity and often lays the groundwork for the final fatal cardiovascular complication, and some reports still list sepsis as the major cause of death.[19]

Acute cholecystitis should be treated surgically early during the acute attack when both the surgeon and the hospital can provide the optimum in diagnosis and care. Cholecystectomy for acute cholecystitis does not lend itself well to occasional surgery but rather should be done as a part of the total care in a hospital with a large volume of biliary tract disease. Once a hospital or a surgeon is committed to the early surgical treatment of acute cholecystitis, it is important to choose the correct operation and to utilize diagnostic methods to improve the diagnostic accuracy, since, as mentioned earlier, the differential diagnosis is not always easy. The patient with right upper quadrant pain, fever, leukocytosis, and a palpable, tender gallbladder presents no problem in diagnosis. A palpable mass representing the gallbladder is probably only demonstrable in half the patients or less. The differential diagnosis between acute cholecystitis and appendicitis, penetrating peptic ulcer, pancreatitis, and sometimes pneumonia may be more cumbersome. It is also important to recognize simple biliary colic without acute cholecystitis, since this does not require early surgery. The differental diagnosis of acute pancreatitis is often the most difficult, particularly since both may coexist. The presence of acute pancreatitis in conjunction with acute cholecystitis requires surgical treatment of the biliary tract disease. Biliary colic with concomitant pancreatitis usually subsides and allows cholecystectomy on an elective basis. The patient with acute pancreatitis not related to biliary tract disease needs to be recognized and separated, since this patient will not be helped by surgery of the biliary tree.

Intravenous cholangiography has been very helpful in the differential diagnosis by permitting opacification of the bile ducts or gallbladder or both and thus on many occasions ruling out the diagnosis of acute cholecystitis. Intravenous cholangiography can be completed in four hours and is carried out while the patient is being treated, examined, and prepared for possible surgery. Visualization of the gallbladder within this time indicates that the cystic duct is not obstructed and thus rules out acute cholecystitis. Pancreatitis usually does not preclude visualization of the biliary tree.[21] Nonvisualization of the gallbladder after four hours indicates cystic duct obstruction and, with other findings, supports the diagnosis of acute cholecystitis. Nonvisualization of both ducts and gallbladder does not aid in the diagnosis of acute cholecystitis except to leave that diagnosis still a possibility. In two series of patients with acute abdominal problems in whom acute cholecystitis was a possible diagnosis, Thorpe[19] found IVC helpful in 85 per cent of his patients, and Chang[4] noted visualization of the biliary tree in 71 per cent of his patients, allowing a decision to be made regarding the presence or absence of acute cholecystitis.

Cholecystostomy

The ideal treatment for acute cholecystitis is early cholecystectomy, that is, removal of the gallbladder during the acute attack. When this is successfully done, the patient is rehabilitated faster and saved future hospitalization for the same disease.

Unfortunately, cholecystectomy is not applicable to all patients with acute cholecystitis, and indeed proper planning of biliary tract surgery demands that the patient with acute cholecystitis be rather carefully selected for cholecystectomy, because the surgery is a major one and is only well tolerated by reasonably healthy people with an acceptable health reserve. The alternative to cholecystectomy in acute cholecystitis is cholecystostomy. Cholecystostomy is a temporary procedure; it does not eradicate the source of the patient's problem, even though removal of the offending calculi is often possible. Cholecystostomy, on the other hand, can be a life-saving procedure for the poor-risk patient and an acceptable way out for the surgeon when he is faced with a technically difficult problem. The following should be considered as indications for cholecystostomy:

1. The poor-risk or aged patient.
2. The patient with a perforated gallbladder and peritonitis.
3. The patient with severe cholecystitis in whom landmarks are obscured and cholecystectomy cannot be safely carried out.

It is inadvisable to set an age limit for cholecystectomy, since some patients in their seventies can tolerate the operation, whereas others in their fifties are unsuitable candidates. On the whole, however, the older the patient, the less likely he is to withstand the rigors of a major procedure.

Technical Aspects

Cholecystostomy may be one of the easiest or one of the most technically difficult operations to perform. The simple cholecystostomy involves the thin patient with an easily palpable gallbladder. In this situation the incision is located over the fundus of the gallbladder, and local anesthesia is easily administered.

The difficult cholecystostomy involves the obese patient with a shrunken gallbladder. In this situation the gallbladder is not palpable, the location of the incision has to be arbitrarily chosen, and the use of local anesthesia is more problematic, since the incision must be larger and deeper and some intra-abdominal exploration is necessary. When the decision for cholecystostomy is made preoperatively, usually based on the patient's general health, it is advisable to plan it in such a way as to constitute the least burden for the patient. Local anesthesia is preferable and is often easily accomplished. The fundus of the gallbladder is exposed through a small incision, and the gallbladder is emptied by a trocar. It is important to obtain a bacterial culture at this time. The gallbladder is rapidly emptied of all accessible stones, and a Malecot catheter of the largest size to be accommodated within the gallbladder is inserted. The catheter is held in place by a pursestring suture. The fundus of the gallbladder is sutured to the posterior rectus fascia and peritoneum. The catheter emerges through a stab wound, and the subcutaneous tissues are drained by a Penrose drain.

The shrunken, acutely inflamed gallbladder, particularly in the obese patient, requires a larger incision. Local anesthesia may still be used. The gallbladder here cannot be sutured to the peritoneum, and both the catheter and the drain should exit through separate stab wounds.

Care of the Cholecystostomy Tube

The tube draining the gallbladder should be left in place for at least ten days. When the cholecystostomy is done as a temporary procedure and an elective cholecystectomy is planned later, the tube is best left in place until the time of the cholecystectomy. The tube may be changed to a smaller size, however, and need not be open for drainage at all times. Cholecystostomy tubes usually stop draining unless a cystic duct obstruction persists and mucus produced by the

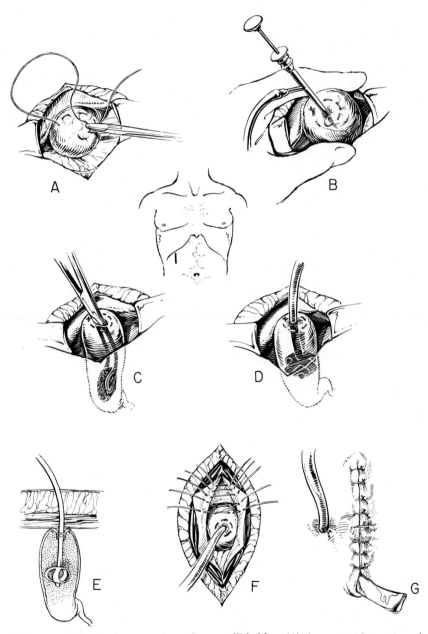

Figure 5–3 Cholecystostomy for a large gallbladder. (*A*) A purse-string suture is placed in the fundus of the gallbladder. (*B*) The gallbladder is decompressed by a trocar. (*C*) The stones are removed. (*D*) A Malecot catheter is in place. (*E and F*) The fundus of the gallbladder is sutured to the peritoneum and posterior rectus fascia. (*G*) The Malecot catheter emerges through a stab wound. A subcutaneous drain is in place. (From Glenn, F., and Thorbjarnarson, B.: The Craft of Surgery. Vol. 2. Boston, Little, Brown and Company, 1964, p. 953.)

gallbladder keeps draining. Continued bile leakage from the tube is discussed in the section on biliary fistulas.

When cholecystostomy is done as a definitive procedure, it is usually permissible to remove the tube within two to three weeks or as soon as drainage has ceased. At times, cholecystostomy tubes may be left in on a permanent basis, only to be changed as needed because of encrustation or deterioration of the tube.

Cholecystectomy

The gallbladder in acute cholecystitis is usually large, tense, purplish in color, and intimately wrapped in omentum and adjacent

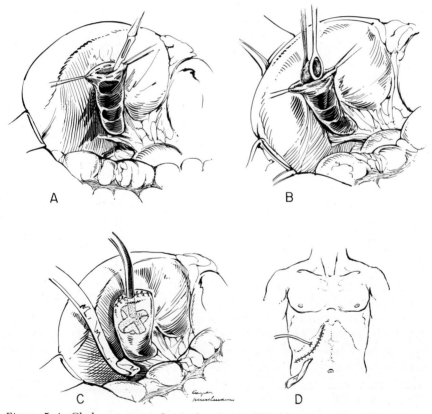

Figure 5–4 Cholecystostomy for a shrunken gallbladder. (*A*) The gallbladder is shrunken and deep under the liver. (*B*) The stones are removed. (*C*) The cholecystostomy is closed around a Malecot catheter. A cigarette drain is placed alongside the gallbladder. (*D*) The catheter and drain emerge through separate stab wounds. (From Glenn, F., and Thorbjarnarson, B.: The Craft of Surgery. Vol. 2. Boston, Little, Brown and Company, 1964, p. 953.)

organs. When the abdomen is entered, some free, straw-colored fluid is usually present and a culture should be taken. The gallbladder itself is often not visible, but a mass covered by omentum is visible and palpable adjacent to and under the right lobe of the liver. The operator is first of all faced with exposing the gallbladder and freeing it from the omentum, transverse colon, duodenum, and antrum of the stomach that have encased it, in order to confine the infection to the right upper quadrant. The attachment between the gallbladder and these organs is reasonably loose for the first two or three days of the attack, and blunt dissection is usually easily accomplished as long as the surgeon finds the correct plane to work in.

Before the removal of the gallbladder is undertaken, the surgeon tries to identify the cystic duct and artery, much as is done in an elective cholecystectomy. Identification of landmarks is sometimes difficult in acute cholecystitis, and one must be prepared to abandon the plan for cholecystectomy in favor of cholecystostomy whenever it becomes apparent that reliable landmarks are hopelessly obscured. Ordinarily, however, as the surgeon proceeds with his dissection, he will encounter the ampulla and soon after see the duodenum. At this time the foramen of Winslow may be identified and the location of the hepatic artery ascertained. The cystic duct lymph node is usually large and firm in acute cholecystitis and may be used as a landmark indicating proximity to the cystic duct—common duct junction. The cystic duct is tentatively identified and a ligature passed around it. The cystic artery is found next, although it is often thrombosed in this situation. A ligature for identification is also passed around the cystic artery.

The question may arise as to whether or not the gallbladder should be decompressed prior to removal. When the organ is of large size, decompression by aspiration is usually necessary to obtain adequate exposure of the porta hepatis. When the gallbladder is of average size, this may not be needed, and when the walls are contracted around the large stones, it is of course not feasible. Except for the identification of the structures in the hepatoduodenal ligament, the removal of the gallbladder from the liver bed is the most critical part of the operation. The problems likely to be encountered involve discovery of perforation into the liver capsule by the disease process and laceration of the liver in the process of removal. The liver is often engorged and its capsule thin and tense in acute cholecystitis. Too much traction on the gallbladder may avulse it from the liver bed, leaving a large, raw area bleeding profusely. Control of this bleeding is difficult, since the capsule is missing and the liver substance does not hold sutures. Avulsion or laceration of the liver is avoided by finding the proper plane for dissection between the gallbladder wall and liver bed. The dissection of the gallbladder or shelling out should start at a safe distance from the liver, at least a centimeter away, and no traction should be exerted until a well-defined plane has been established. This dissection starts at the fundus and proceeds toward the ampulla. Vessels from the liver to the gallbladder and the posterior division of the cystic artery are divided and secured as they are encountered. In difficult circumstances it is worth remembering that it is not necessary to remove the entire wall of the gallbladder. As long as the mucosa is removed, the surgeon is accomplishing his objective. When the gallbladder is entered in the liver bed, either because of a perforation or through surgical trauma, it is advisable to establish a new plane farther down on the gallbladder and to work proximally toward the perforation to avoid leaving part of the mucosa behind. The inflammatory reaction in acute cholecystitis is usually most marked around the fundus and body of the gallbladder, and when it has been possible to identify the cystic duct before starting the removal, the operation becomes easier as one approaches the common duct. At all times the surgeon must be in contact with the gallbladder wall during its removal from the liver and while freeing it from the ampulla. The handling of the acutely inflamed gallbladder during removal thus differs quite a bit from that during elective cholecystectomy. It may not be possible to place clamps on the gallbladder for retraction, since the wall has lost its substance and the instruments cut through. The need to stay in the correct plane to avoid liver damage and to avoid encroachment on the hepatic artery and hepatic duct may dictate opening the gallbladder, evacuating stones, and placing a finger inside it for guidance in the dissection of these critical areas.

CHOLESTEROSIS OF THE GALLBLADDER

Cholesterosis of the gallbladder indicates accumulation of lipid in the epithelial cells and macrophages in the subepithelial layer of the gallbladder wall. Clinically the condition is referred to as "strawberry gallbladder." The accumulation of the lipid is not associated with cholecystitis but apparently is related to a high concentration of cholesterol in the gallbladder bile. Pathologically the lipid accumulates in the wall of the gallbladder and may occupy the villi of the lining of the gallbladder, forming a polyp. This polyp is seen on cholecystograms as a fixed filling defect; it may be detached and form a nidus for stone formation or, more often, only form debris in the gallbladder that may give rise to pain and colic as it is evacuated through the cystic duct.

Cholesterosis occurs in both men and women and may give rise to symptoms similar to those of gallstones. The diagnosis is difficult unless fixed filling defects are seen on the cholecystogram. Sometimes there is evidence of overconcentration of the dye in the gall-

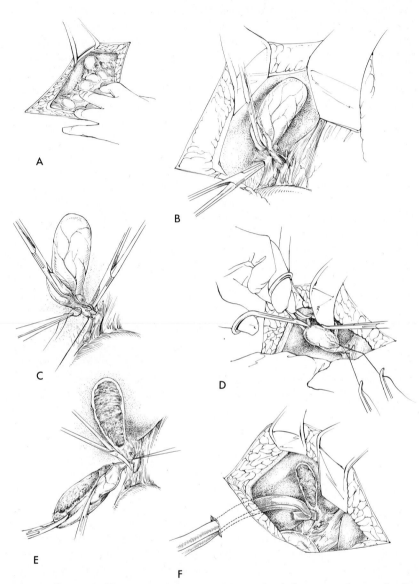

Figure 5–5 Cholecystectomy technique. (A) A subcostal incision brings the liver edge and the gallbladder into view. The transverse colon is located under the liver and the gallbladder. (B) The cystic duct can best be approached from behind rather than anteriorly through Calot's triangle. Once the cystic duct has been identified posteriorly or in the edge of the hepatoduodenal ligament, identification of the artery and the common duct becomes much easier. (C) The cystic duct and cystic artery are both temporarily occluded with a ligature of silk. (D) The gallbladder is dissected out of its liver bed from the fundus down. A retractor inside the liver bed aids in the exposure. (E) The cystic artery has been ligated and divided. The cystic duct is being divided after exposing the common duct above and below the juncture. (F) Two Penrose drains are placed through a stab wound down to the cystic duct.

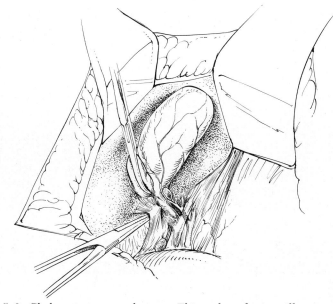

Figure 5–6 Cholecystectomy technique. This enlarged view illustrates some of the landmarks the surgeon can use in orienting himself during cholecystectomy. The hepatic artery is farthest to the right in the hepatoduodenal ligament and can usually be palpated, placing the bile duct immediately lateral to the artery. The lymph node in the angle between the duodenum and the common bile duct is seen. This is often a prominent feature which aids in alerting the surgeon to the proximity of the common bile duct. The cystic duct lymph node is seen between the two branching divisions of the cystic artery. This node again tells the surgeon that the cystic artery is near and that the common bile duct is not too far medially.

bladder on cholecystography, and this may indicate the possibility of cholesterosis. Duodenal drainage may show large amounts of cholesterol crystals and does aid in diagnosis. At surgery, the gallbladder with cholesterosis is thin-walled but of bright blue color. The cholesterol deposits cannot be palpated because of their softness.

Cholesterosis of the gallbladder may cause symptoms similar to those of gallstones, and these symptoms are relieved by cholecystectomy. We do not have information relating to the frequency of cholesterosis, but it is commonly seen at autopsy. Asymptomatic cholesterosis is not an indication for cholecystectomy.

ADENOMYOMATOSIS OF THE GALLBLADDER AND ASCHOFF-ROKITANSKY SINUSES

Adenomyomatosis is probably a distinct entity from true Aschoff-Rokitansky sinuses.[33,34] Adenomyomatosis is a congenital anomaly

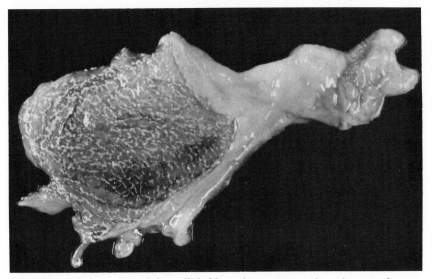

Figure 5–7 Cholesterosis of the gallbladder. The picture is that of a typical strawberry gallbladder. The villi of the gallbladder mucosa are distended with lipids and give the gallbladder its speckled yellow color when opened up. The villi may become large enough to be seen on cholecystograms as fixed filling defects. The lipid-laden villi may become sequestered and fall into the gallbladder, causing colic and symptoms typical of cholelithiasis. Symptomatic cholesterosis is an indication for cholecystectomy.

that involves the fundus of the gallbladder and presents grossly as a palpable mass with normal serosal covering. When the tumor or mass is transected, it is found honeycombed with cystic spaces that may or may not communicate with the gallbladder lumen. Aschoff-Rokitansky sinuses, on the other hand, are acquired and are almost never seen in young people. The normal gallbladder mucosa sits directly on the muscularis without an intervening submucosa. Aschoff-Rokitansky sinuses represent outpouchings of the gallbladder mucosa that insinuate themselves between the muscle bundles and may work their way to the serosal surface. In this way they are false diverticula similar to a Zenker's diverticulum in the esophagus.

Both adenomyomatosis and Aschoff-Rokitansky sinuses represent pathologic states and are usually symptomatic. Radiologically, adenomyomatosis is demonstrated as a filling defect in the fundus of the gallbladder, or the cystic spaces are filled with the dye and demonstrate the honeycombed appearance. The Aschoff-Rokitansky sinuses project outside the lumen of the gallbladder and, when numerous, may look like a row of beads surrounding the organ. The cause of the Aschoff-Rokitansky sinuses is probably excessive pressure within the gallbladder and may be related to chronic inflammation and difficulty evacuating bile through the cystic duct. Both adenomyomatosis and

Aschoff-Rokitansky sinuses involve formation of closed or semiclosed diverticula and spaces outside the gallbladder lumen. In these spaces the components of the bile have an opportunity to precipitate and desiccate, thus forming concretions. Both conditions are usually associated with symptoms and are an indication for cholecystectomy.

CHOLEDOCHOLITHIASIS

It may be estimated that, of all persons in the United States with gallstones, 12 per cent have calculi in the ductal system outside the gallbladder.[41] It is assumed by surgeons that most stones residing within the common bile duct have been formed in the gallbladder and have passed from there into the bile duct. On rare occasions (less than 1 per cent), stones may be found in the bile duct without evidence of stones in the gallbladder.[46] A varied situation is found in other areas of the world, particularly in the Far East, where calculi in the common duct are found quite commonly without stones in the gallbladder. The gallstones found in the common duct among persons residing in Western countries usually have the same composition as stones in

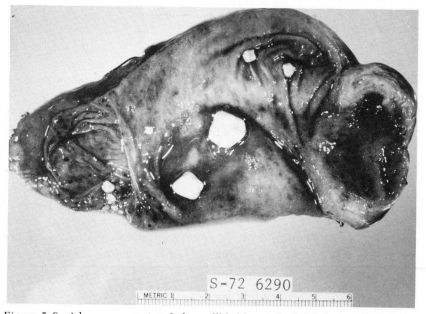

S-72 6290

METRIC | 2| 3| 4| 5| 6|

Figure 5–8 Adenomyomatosis of the gallbladder and cholelithiasis. The adenomyomatosis is seen as a thick-walled, honeycomb-like area resembling a tumor in the fundus of the gallbladder, which is at the right side of the photograph. Adenomyomatosis often coexists with cholelithiasis but may be symptomatic without cholelithiasis, in which case symptoms are also relieved by cholecystectomy.

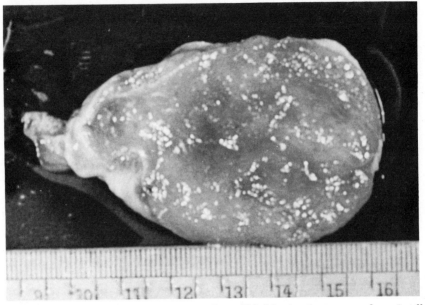

Figure 5–9   Aschoff-Rokitansky sinuses. The gallbladder has been opened up. Small elevations on the surface indicate Aschoff-Rokitansky sinuses containing calcareous debris. Stone formation may start within the enclosed spaces of the Aschoff-Rokitansky sinuses, and debris from the sinuses may form the nidus of further stone formation within the gallbladder itself.

the gallbladder that are primarily made up of cholesterol. In the Far East, stones found in the ductal system and particularly in the intrahepatic branches of the hepatic ducts are usually composed of bile pigment and contents of bile other than cholesterol and are thus often classified as inflammatory stones. In Taiwan men and women are equally affected by intrahepatic stones, and the age incidence is much lower than that involving common duct stones in the Western countries.[54] The highest incidence of intrahepatic stones in Taiwan is in the age group between 20 and 30. Also, only about a third of the patients with intrahepatic stones have calculi in the gallbladder at the same time. The cause of the intrahepatic stones in the population of the Far East is not known. In some areas of the Far East, they are attributed to infestation with liver fluke, but obviously this is not the entire explanation, since the disease is common in Taiwan where liver flukes do not exist.

Symptoms

The symptoms of choledocholithiasis are pain, jaundice, and fever, but they vary considerably. In a large series of patients coming to surgery for common duct stones, pain was found in 91 per cent of the patients, jaundice in 76 per cent, and fever in 29 per cent.[42] Often these symptoms overlap, and some patients may have all three symptoms, whereas others have only one. The type of pain in choledocholithiasis also varies considerably. Most often it is the crampy, colicky, midepigastric pain with some radiation to the back. On other occasions, however, it may not radiate, and on occasion it is described as a girdlelike pain, particularly when the stone is impacted in the ampulla of Vater. The pain distribution in choledocholithiasis also depends to some extent on the organs affected. When pancreatitis is superimposed on the biliary obstruction, the pain often shifts to the left upper quadrant or even to the left shoulder, and the element of back pain may become even more prominent. There are occasions in which pain is absent and the only signs or symptoms are those of jaundice or fever. The stone that blocks the ampulla of Vater and remains impacted usually leads to progressive and unremittent jaundice and thus may simulate the onset of the painless progressive jaundice of a malignant tumor. More commonly, the stones do not cause a complete obstruction. The stone may move back and forth and obstruct the bile duct intermittently, causing periodic attacks of pain and jaundice; with superimposed infection, fever and chills become a part of the picture.

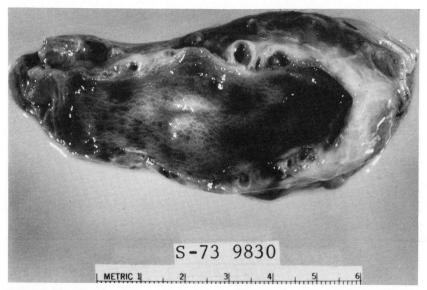

S-73 9830

Figure 5-10 Chronic cholecystitis and Aschoff-Rokitansky sinuses. The gallbladder does not contain any calculi, but the wall is thickened and the Aschoff-Rokitansky sinuses are easily seen in the cut edge of the specimen. Aschoff-Rokitansky sinuses may be diagnosed radiologically and, when associated with symptoms, are an indication for cholecystectomy.

Physical Examination

Physical examination of patients with choledocholithiasis is rarely characteristic in any way. They are often jaundiced, and there is often tenderness over an enlarged liver when infection is present. The gallbladder is usually not palpable unless a concomitant empyema, hydrops, or acute cholecystitis is present, since chronic inflammatory changes in the gallbladder prevent it from enlarging and becoming palpable, contrary to the rule in obstruction from malignant tumors.

Bile Duct Size and Pathologic Anatomy

The common bile duct is the segment of the extrahepatic bile ducts extending from the junction of the cystic and hepatic ducts down to its entrance into the duodenum. The length of the common duct varies considerably, depending on the insertion of the cystic duct into the hepatic duct.[48] The average length is estimated at 7.5 cm. The extremes in variation would occur when the cystic duct enters the right hepatic duct (which rarely happens), in which case there is no common hepatic duct, and when the cystic duct enters the ampulla of Vater in the retroduodenal area, in which case there is no true common bile duct. These variations are extremely rare, however, and in over 75 per cent of cases the length of the common bile duct is close to 7.5 cm. The outer diameter of the common bile duct varies between 4 and 12 mm[48] and averages 7.39 mm. The diameter of the bile duct increases with the patient's age, but there is no relation between the caliber of the duct and the size or weight of the patient. The thickness of the wall of the common duct varies from 0.8 to 1.5 mm.

With obstruction or infection or both, the thickness, diameter, and length of the common bile duct change considerably. With prolonged obstruction, the diameter of the duct may be 12 cm or more, and when this obstruction is due to stones and accompanied by infection, the duct wall becomes thickened and indurated. Once stones are located within the common bile duct, they inevitably lead to progressive change. This change is affected by both local pressure on the wall of the duct and intermittent, varying degrees of obstruction, leading to thickening of the wall and dilatation of the duct, as well as secondary changes in the liver. The size of the common duct and the thickness of the common duct wall vary directly with the duration of intermittent obstruction, and the wall is thicker and the diameter of the lumen is larger the more intermittent and long-standing the obstruction is. It should be remembered that a common duct that becomes obstructed and remains obstructed from a stone never reaches the size of one that has intermittent episodes of obstruction over long periods of time before surgical correction is undertaken.

Chronic intermittent or acute common duct obstruction from a stone affects the liver in many ways. Acute suppurative cholangitis, which will be described in detail later, may be superimposed on ascending cholangitis. Liver abscesses may form, which are usually multiple and small rather than large and discrete. Intermittent obstruction without acute purulent infection results in fibrosis and scarring of the liver substance, creating portal fibrosis and the condition of biliary cirrhosis. The surface of the liver is at first finely granular and later irregular and hobnailed, but the surface is always more finely nodular than in Laennec's cirrhosis. In the early stages of biliary cirrhosis, the liver is often enlarged and may remain so; in the later stages, it may shrink and diminish in size as increased fibrosis takes place in the liver parenchyma. Also in the later stages portal hypertension becomes evident; the spleen is then found to be enlarged, and the veins in the portal system are large, tortuous, and distended. In this situation the surgical approach to the porta hepatis for relief of bile duct obstruction becomes hazardous and technically difficult. The bile duct obstructed by a malignant neoplasm is usually free from infection and thus remains thin-walled and blue without induration and does not reach the gigantic size sometimes seen in intermittent obstruction over a period of years by a stone.

The surgeon's decision as to when to explore or examine the inside of a common bile duct during surgery for biliary tract disease may be based on many different observations.[36,38,41,45] The first and most obvious reason for common duct exploration is the presence of jaundice at the time of surgery. A second reason is palpation of a calculus within the bile duct during surgery or the demonstration of a stone within the duct prior to surgery by intravenous cholangiography. A history of jaundice or intermittent jaundice in the past is a compelling reason for exploring the common bile duct or at least obtaining a good cholangiogram during surgery. A large and thick-walled common bile duct deserves exploration, since these findings are usually secondary to obstruction and infection in the past. A history of recurring attacks of pancreatitis in conjunction with biliary tract disease and the finding of an indurated or thickened pancreas at the time of surgery for biliary tract disease are indications for common duct exploration. The presence of multiple small stones in the gallbladder, particularly with a patent cystic duct, would indicate the possibility that some of these small stones have passed into the common bile duct, and exploration should be carried out. A patient with a cholecystoenteric fistula should always undergo common duct exploration, since the presence of an open fistula may indicate obstruction at the distal end of the common duct. The same may be said when operations are carried out for a retained cystic duct stump, particularly when stones are found in the stump at exploration.

Intraoperative Cholangiography and Manometry

An adjunct to exploration of the common bile duct is the intraoperative cholangiogram, which often may be done through the cystic duct at the time of cholecystectomy or through a needle that punctures the common bile duct. Many surgeons believe that an intraoperative cholangiogram should be done each time a gallbladder is removed for a stone, irrespective of the presence or absence of classic indications for common duct exploration.

The need for improved methods both in common duct exploration for stones and in adjunct measures for discovering stones in the common duct is obvious, since 2 to 4 per cent of patients undergoing surgery for calculi will come to reoperation at a later date for retained calculi within the common duct.[41]

Although most surgeons adhere to similar indications relating to common bile duct exploration, the number of patients undergoing common duct exploration varies considerably among different hospitals. The incidence of stones recovered from common duct exploration also varies considerably. It is important to limit the exploration of the common duct whenever possible, since there is universal agreement that the addition of common duct exploration to cholecystectomy increases the morbidity and mortality.[41,46] On the other hand, it is also important not to leave behind stones, since these are certain sources of future complications for the patient. At the New York Hospital[41] 15 per cent of patients undergoing surgery for chronic biliary tract disease undergo common duct exploration on the basis of the indications mentioned earlier. Among these patients, stones are found in 8.8 per cent. In the same hospital the same indications are used for exploration of the common bile duct during surgery for acute cholecystitis; 13 per cent of the patients undergoing surgery for this disorder have undergone common duct exploration in the past, and stones were found in 7.5 per cent. In other institutions[36] common duct explorations are carried out in up to 42 per cent of patients with chronic cholecystitis, and stones are found in 16 per cent.

Other surgeons report the use of biliary tract pressures during surgery to help them decide whether or not to explore the common bile duct.[56] The upper limits of normal biliary pressure measured through the cystic duct are from 15 to 16 cm of saline above the level of the common bile duct, and White et al. believe that a pressure above 16 cm is reliable evidence of an abnormality in the ductal

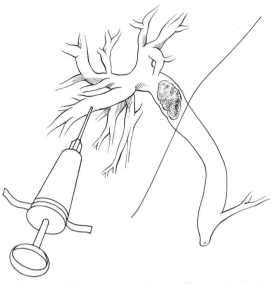

Figure 5–11 Transhepatic cholangiogram. The needle is passed through the edge of the liver into a branch of the hepatic duct. This method is helpful in delineating high-lying tumors or strictures not accessible through the hepatoduodenal ligament.

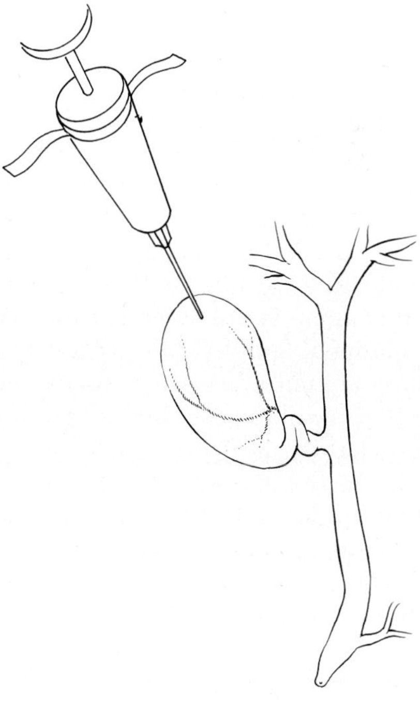

Figure 5–12 Cholecystocho-langiogram. This method is rarely helpful during opera-tion. It does not allow clear vis-ualization of small gallbladder stones, and the contrast material may not pass through the cystic duct to opacify the common duct. Its main use is to delineate a normal biliary tree.

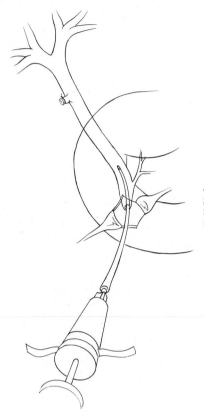

Figure 5–13 Duodenotomy and retro-grade cholangiography. Difficult to do but may be needed when bile duct cannot be identified in hepatoduodenal ligament.

system. They feel, however, that this test must be used in con-junction with cholangiography, since there are both false-positive and false-negative results in the use of manometry alone. These same authors also believe that a cholangiogram alone gives up to 6 per cent false-negative results, with some false-positive results, and indicate that this alone is not sufficient to make an accurate diagnosis. Opera-tive cholangiography can obviously be a very important adjunct in locating common bile duct stones and an aid in the decision whether or not to explore the bile duct during surgery for calculi.[46] This method has its shortcomings, however, as does any diagnostic method, and the help it gives relates directly to the time and effort the surgeon and the radiologist put into it in each individual institution. When intraoperative cholangiography is done properly with good technical assistance and good equipment, it is of the utmost help to the surgeon.

Some of the reasons for failure of the operative cholangiogram have recently been well described.[43] The authors reviewed the findings of 302 patients who had T-tube cholangiography following

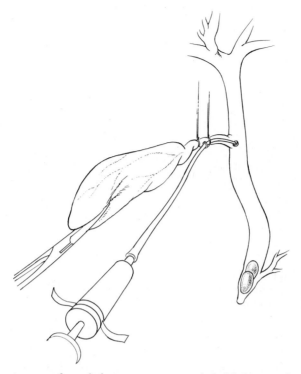

Figure 5–14 A cystic duct cholangiogram is very helpful for visualization of the common duct during cholecystectomy. It is virtually free of errors due to introduction of air bubbles. There is no danger of bile leak postoperatively, since the cystic duct is ligated distal to the area where the catheter is introduced.

Figure 5–15 A needle cholangiogram is done when the gallbladder is missing or when the cystic duct cannot be used for introduction of a catheter. The needle is of a fine caliber with a fairly blunt end and is bent to prevent penetration of the posterior wall of the duct. A needle cholangiogram prior to choledochotomy avoids the introduction of air bubbles and allows an accurate estimate of the number of calculi present.

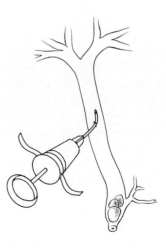

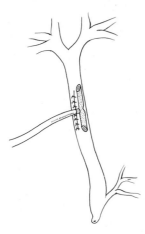

Figure 5–16 The T-tube cholangiogram is an essential step following removal of common duct stones. It may, however, be inaccurate unless extraordinary care is taken not to introduce air bubbles that may simulate stones.

common duct exploration before they were discharged from the hospital. The findings were that in 41 patients, or over 14 per cent, stones had been left behind in the common bile duct. Whereas a 14 per cent incidence of retained stones is certainly high, the reasons for this are well brought out in this article. One of the common causes for retained stones following common duct exploration is overreliance on and overconfidence in the cholangiography. The x-ray technician has to know the proper exposure time, which is related to the patient's size and shape, and there must be cooperation between the surgeon, the anesthesiologist, and the x-ray technician in obtaining the exposure at the proper moment when the patient is in apnea. The ordinary contrast material is used at 50 per cent strength. In large, dilated ducts this strength can obscure smaller stones; the larger the duct, the more dilute the material should be. The ductal system may be incompletely filled on the x-ray film; in order to obtain complete filling of the ductal system, particularly of the intrahepatic radices, it may be necessary to tilt the patient in Trendelenburg's position to make the intrahepatic duct dependent and more easily filled. On occasion, it may be necessary to occlude the terminal portion of the common duct to obtain a complete filling of the intrahepatic duct. Attention has been paid to the positioning of the patient, since superimposition of parts of the ductal system, and perhaps superimposition of elements of the spine, may be misinterpreted as stones or filling defects.

The indication for common bile duct exploration thus has to be each surgeon's individual decision. The safety of relying on the old and established criteria of (1) jaundice past or present, (2) palpable stones in the common duct, (3) enlarged or thick-walled duct, (4) large cystic duct with small stones in the gallbladder, (5) recurrent pancreatitis or evidence of chronic pancreatitis at surgery, (6) biliary enteric fistula, and (7) cystic duct remnant with or without stones has been well established. Adjuncts to these are the preoperative intravenous cholangiogram[39] and the intraoperative cystic duct or needle cholangiogram. None of the indications or adjuncts is absolute or infallible, but by judicious use of all or some, depending on the circumstances and particularly the quality of intraoperative x-rays, the patient will be best served.

Retained Common Bile Duct Stones

Tubes placed in the common bile duct for decompression after exploration for stones should not be removed until a cholangiogram has demonstrated the ductal system to be patent and free of calculi. The postoperative cholangiogram should usually be performed on the ninth or tenth postoperative day; it is usually quite accurate, since it is performed in the radiologist's domain where all proper equipment and technical help are available. The most troublesome aspect of these tube cholangiograms is the occasional introduction of air bubbles, which tend to simulate stones, into the biliary tree. Usually the air bubbles are easily detected and separated from true stones, since they are usually several in number and inconsistent, but always perfectly round. The stones, on the other hand, are consistent and usually not of a perfectly round shape. The risk of introducing air bubbles may be minimized by the following maneuver. The tube is held and allowed to fill from the bile duct until it is overflowing. The tube is then occluded by a clamp, and the dye used for the cholangiogram is injected from a syringe through a needle stuck through the wall of the tube. Once a retained stone or stones is demonstrated in the bile duct, a decision has to be made as to how to proceed. Obviously removal of the drainage tube with a stone remaining should not be advocated, since either a biliary fistula or jaundice might result. There are several choices at present, but none is entirely satisfactory. Personally I prefer to reoperate on the patient, particularly when his general health is good. This operation should be done when the patient is in the optimum condition but may well be done within days of discovery of the stone.

Intracholedochal drip of heparin[40] and, more recently, the administration of chenodeoxycholic acid have been recommended for dissolution of the stone. Both methods have not been adequately proved to be universally acceptable. The extraction of residual stones by passing baskets through the tract of the drainage tube has received much attention and is a possible answer in cases in which the drainage tube has been of sufficient size to permit passage of the basket.[35,37,49,50] Although retrieval of stones by a basket has worked well in selected instances, it is probably not the ideal method, and each patient will have to be evaluated on his own merits.

Exploration of the Common Bile Duct

The incision of choice for operations on the gallbladder and common duct is the right subcostal one, extending across the midline when need be. The reason for choosing the subcostal incision is that it gives easy access to the liver edge. The approach to the common bile duct in difficult situations is to follow the liver edge and under-surface of the liver medially to the porta hepatis. During this approach the omentum, transverse colon, duodenum, and pylorus are encountered and freed from the undersurface of the liver. The duct is located in the lateral edge of the hepatoduodenal ligament and may be located by following the cystic duct when the gallbladder is still present. When the gallbladder has been removed, the common duct is most easily approached along the lateral border of the duodenum toward the porta hepatis. A lymph node is usually present in the angle between the common duct and the duodenum, and this alerts the operator. Once the duodenum has been exposed to the pylorus, the foramen of Winslow should be accessible, and palpation of the hepatoduodenal ligament identifies the hepatic artery. The common duct is located between the free edge of the hepatoduodenal ligament and the hepatic artery. When cholecystectomy has been done, the stump of the cystic duct may often be found and will aid in orientation. The stump is usually about 3 cm above the upper border of the duodenum. The surface of the duct is often identified by thin venules in its outer coat and possibly by a blue or green color when it is sufficiently thin-walled. At times extensive adhesions and scarring may make identification of the duct difficult, and aspiration with a fine-bore needle will often aid in proper location. When difficulty has been encountered in identifying the common duct and it is finally located by aspiration, it is advisable to do a cholangiogram through the needle to further identify its course and condition.

The duct is opened lengthwise between stay sutures for exploration. The length of the choledochotomy depends on the diameter of the duct. It must at least be close to 2 cm to allow the use of instruments for exploration. The largest ducts should be opened much more widely so that a finger can be introduced for palpation. A cholangiogram done through a needle or through the cystic duct makes it possible to obtain an x-ray free of the air bubbles that often confound the surgeon when doing T-tube cholangiograms. The initial x-ray may then allow the surgeon to count the stones residing within the common duct and know beforehand how many he must retrieve.

The method and modes of retrieving stones from the bile duct are almost as many as there are surgeons doing biliary tract surgery. The method described here is simple, but in large series of patients in the hands of many different surgeons, it has resulted in overlooked stones or reformed stones in only 3 to 4 per cent. Once the bile duct is open, a culture should be done of its contents. The most productive instrument for retrieving stones from the lower common duct is the pituitary spoon. One should use the largest spoon that fits the duct initially, progressing to the smaller ones. The duct should be explored systematically, usually starting with the lower part toward the duodenum. During removal of stones from the ducts, it may be helpful to place a small gauze pad tied to a string in the upper or lower end of the choledochotomy in order to avoid stones migrating from one part of the duct to the other. Once the ducts have been evacuated with the spoons and stone forceps, irrigation is carried out using saline. Soft rubber catheters are used and passed into individual hepatic ducts, as well as into the lower common duct.

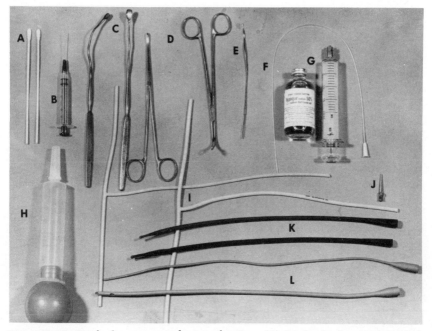

Figure 5-17 Tools for common duct exploration. (A) Swabs for bacteriologic culture. (B) Small (2 ml) syringe with No. 21 needle for aspiration of bile. (C) Malleable pituitary scoops of varying sizes. (D) Stone forceps, straight and curved. (E) Silver probe for probing and locating pancreatic duct. (F) Cholangiocatheter for cystic duct cholangiogram. (G) 50% Hypaque and syringe for cholangiography. (H) Bulb syringe for irrigation. (I) T-tubes in varying sizes from No. 8 to No. 20. (J) Adaptor for small bore T-tubes. (K) Flexible hollow bougies, in varying sizes from No. 8 to No. 26, for passage through ampulla of Vater. (L) Red rubber catheters for irrigation.

After the stones have been removed, the surgeons must demonstrate patency of the ampulla of Vater. This may be done with a soft rubber catheter, but more often semirigid bougies of graduated sizes are used, and bougies the diameter of a lead pencil should pass into the duodenum. With the bougie in place in the duodenum, the duct is again palpated; remaining stones are often felt on the bougie and may thus be removed. The use of rigid instruments for passage through the ampulla of Vater is sometimes risky, since one of the serious complications of common duct exploration is perforation of the duct, particularly in its intrapancreatic duodenal position. When patency of the ampulla of Vater cannot be demonstrated, it becomes incumbent upon the surgeon to do a duodenotomy, as described elsewhere.

Following common bile duct exploration, drainage through either a T-tube or a straight catheter should be instituted. While it is true that, on occasion, the bile duct can be closed primarily without drainage, this is not to be recommended for universal acceptance. The T-tube used is notched and should fit loosely in the bile duct. The choledochotomy is closed around the tube by fine chromic catgut sutures and is reinforced by silk sutures that do not penetrate the ductal wall. Common duct drainage by a straight tube is best accomplished through the cystic duct, with the tube pointing distally, and thorough closure of the choledochotomy used for the exploration. Tubes for decompression of the common duct should be placed judiciously. The ends should not be too long and must not impinge on the ampulla of Vater or be too close to the bifurcation of the hepatic duct. A cholangiogram should be done at the end of the operation, as described earlier. Common bile duct drains and drains following cholecystectomy should emerge through separate stab wounds away from the main incision. A T-tube is allowed to drain dependently postoperatively. On the ninth or tenth postoperative day, the T-tube may be attached to a manometer to determine the resistance at the sphincter of Oddi. Pressures of 20 cm or less of water are normal. A cholangiogram is done the day after determination of the intraductal pressures, and if the x-ray is normal, the tube can be removed. The tube should not be removed on the day of the cholangiogram, since rarely but occasionally cholangitis requiring continued drainage may follow the x-ray.

Ancillary Procedures in Common Duct Exploration

It is clear that the problem of common duct stones is not solved as long as 3 to 4 per cent of calculi are overlooked during surgery and may require secondary procedures. Several measures have been advo-

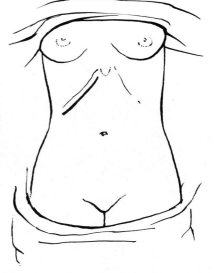

Figure 5–18 Exploration of the common duct. The incision preferred for exploration of the common bile duct is a right subcostal incision two finger breadths below the right costal margin, extending from the midline obliquely across the rectus muscle. The incision can be extended across the linea alba and also out into the oblique muscles if need be.

cated in addition to the well known one of high-quality operative cholangiography. Recently, the filling of the bile duct with plasma clot that envelops the stones and allows easier extraction has been described.[48] Endoscopy has been used to locate both stones and tumor within the duct.[51,52] Special catheters with small inflatable

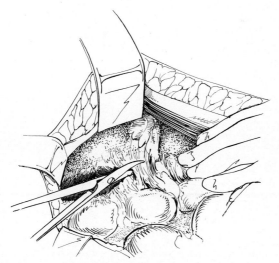

Figure 5–19 The common duct is approached from the lateral side, identifying the edge of the liver and dissecting the transverse colon, the pylorus, and the antrum of the stomach away from the right lobe of the liver.

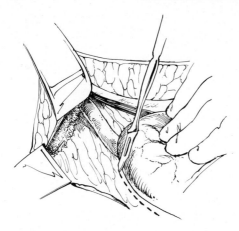

Figure 5-20 To gain access to the lower end of the common bile duct, the peritoneal reflection from the duodenum is incised, and the duodenum together with the head of the pancreas and lower end of the bile duct is rotated over to the patient's left side—the so-called Kocher's maneuver.

balloons may be passed up and down the duct in order to deliver the stones on withdrawal of the inflated balloon.[44-47] All these methods have something to offer and deserve adequate trial. The danger with the balloon-tipped catheter is that the balloon catches at the narrowed part of the junctures of the intrahepatic ducts, and disruption of the smaller duct may occur when too much force is used.

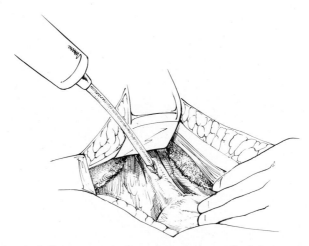

Figure 5-21 A cholangiogram is done through the wall of the common bile duct with a needle attached to a syringe. The use of the needle in a cholangiogram avoids introduction of air and may give accurate information as to the number of stones residing within the common bile duct.

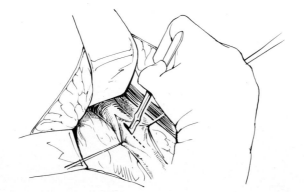

Figure 5–22 The common bile duct is opened between stay sutures. The incision is usually located opposite the cystic duct. When there are plans for a possible chole-dochoduodenostomy, the incision should be lower down, at the upper border of the duodenum, and perhaps transverse or oblique in nature.

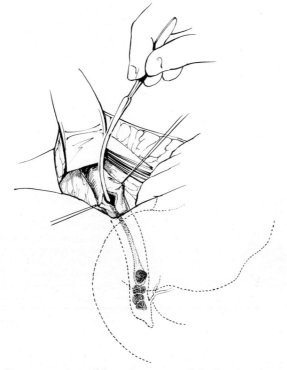

Figure 5–23 Stones are removed from the common bile duct by using pituitary spoons of various sizes. The largest spoon accommodated in a duct is usually the best one for the initial removal of stones. Straight and curved forceps are also sometimes help-ful in removing stones from the extremes of the bile duct.

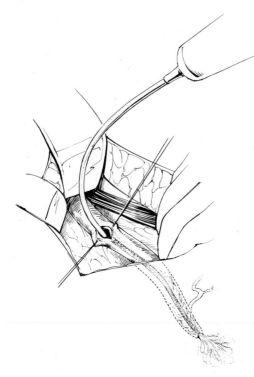

Figure 5–24 After all palpable stones are removed, the bile duct is thoroughly irrigated both distally and proximally within the hepatic ducts. This may flush out gravel or mud and small stones that otherwise are not retrieved.

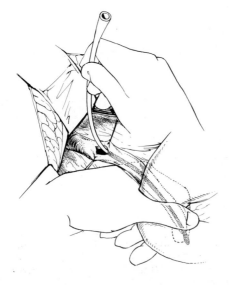

Figure 5–25 Catheters and bougies of increasing size are passed through the ampulla of Vater to test its patency. A tight sphincter of Oddi associated with common bile duct stones indicates the need for duodenotomy and sphincteroplasty to promote better drainage. By passing a bougie through the ampulla of Vater and palpating the duct with the bougie inside it, the operator can feel retained stones against the bougie.

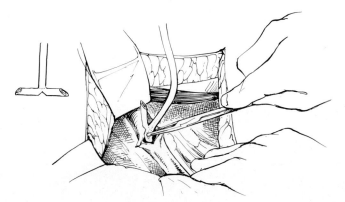

Figure 5–26 The common bile duct is drained by a T-tube following the exploration. The T-tube should be of the smallest size adequate for proper drainage of the duct. Only rarely is a T-tube bigger than No. 14 French necessary for common bile duct drainage. The arms of the T-tube within the duct should be short, so that they do not impinge on the walls of the duct at the bifurcation of the hepatic ducts or down near the ampulla of Vater, causing obstruction of the tube. A triangular piece is cut out of the T-tube at the junction of the arms; this makes removal of the T-tube easier postoperatively.

ACUTE OBSTRUCTIVE CHOLANGITIS

Acute obstructive cholangitis is a rare but serious type of purulent infection in the biliary tree; it usually occurs proximal to an obstructing common duct stone but rarely is superimposed on obstruction of a neoplastic nature.

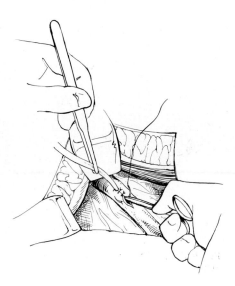

Figure 5–27 The choledochotomy is closed around the T-tube using fine chromic catgut sutures that go through all layers of the bile duct. This closure should be water-tight. A cholangiogram is performed through the tube prior to abdominal wound closure to demonstrate patency of the bile duct and absence of filling defects, indicating that all calculi have been removed.

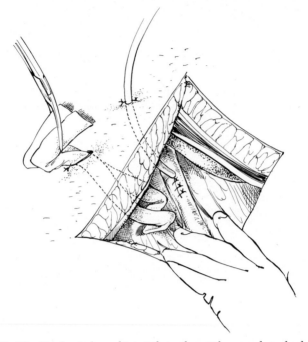

Figure 5–28   The T-tube is brought out through a stab wound, and adequate slack is left in the tube inside the abdomen to prevent dislocation when the patient wakes up and recovers his muscle tone. The drains are brought out through a separate stab wound; both drains and T-tube are secured at the skin level to prevent accidental removal.

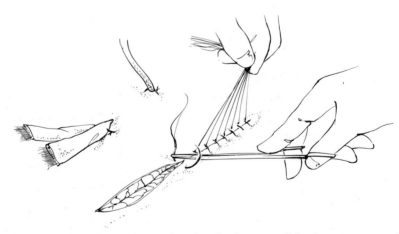

Figure 5–29   The abdominal wound is closed in layers, and the drains are secured in place.

Symptoms

The symptoms of acute obstructive cholangitis are similar to those of common bile duct stones with obstruction and jaundice. The patients are usually past middle age, and many have had known gallbladder disease for a period of time. The symptoms are characterized by acute illness and abdominal pain localized to the right upper quadrant and sometimes to the scapular area. There is rising jaundice, fever, and chills. The triad of jaundice, pain, and fever does not signify much more than acute cholangitis. The diagnosis of acute obstructive cholangitis can only be made in this situation when, added to the three commonly known symptoms, there is evidence of central nervous system involvement and hypotension.[62]

Diagnosis

The diagnosis of acute obstructive cholangitis is based on the history and findings described above. The temperature is usually high, and the fever and chills are quite pronounced. Blood tests are not always helpful. The white blood cell count does not always rise significantly, but there is a pronounced shift to the younger forms of the polymorphonuclear leukocytes. There is tenderness and often rebound tenderness in the right upper quadrant; the liver may be enlarged and tender. The gallbladder may be palpable and tender. The serum bilirubin is usually significantly elevated, and there is a rise in the alkaline phosphatase and a concomitant rise in the serum transaminase during the acute episode. It must be realized, however, that some of the most acutely ill patients may not yet have developed clinical jaundice when they are first seen. Blood cultures are usually positive, showing growth of organisms of the same type as those cultured from the bile at operation, usually gram-negative and enteric organisms. The specific findings in acute obstructive cholangitis are hypotension, shock, and mental confusion.

Etiology

Acute obstructive cholangitis is a virulent type of the common ascending cholangitis seen in biliary tract disease. The specific changes in this variety of cholangitis seem to be based on the overwhelming bacteremia and sepsis originating from the bile ducts. The prerequisite for development of the syndrome seems to be development of high pressures inside the common bile duct, and the pressures inside the duct probably need to be elevated above the maximum secretory pressure of the liver. Huang has shown that positive blood cultures can be obtained in animals with cholangitis when the pressures in the bile duct are raised to above the normal maximum secretory pressure of the liver.[61] He also has demonstrated that bacteria can be cultured both from the lymph and from the blood of these animals at 70 per cent of the maximal hepatic secretory pressure and are found in the peripheral blood at slightly higher pressure. Based on this experimental evidence, it seems that bacteria regurgitate into the circulation from the bile duct. How the high pressures are developed inside the biliary tree is not entirely clear, but it may be through massive proliferation of the bacteria within the bile duct and through the development of large amounts of pus within a short period of time.

Treatment

The treatment of acute obstructive cholangitis is surgical. Patients admitted with cholangitis who fail to respond to the initial treatment with antibiotics and who then develop the symptoms and signs of mental confusion and hypotension should be explored without delay. At operation, a large, thick-walled, edematous, tense common bile duct is usually found, and bile and pus under pressure spurt from the duct as soon as an incision is made. The important part of the surgery is establishment of adequate drainage from the common bile duct. Depending on the condition of the patient, the common duct may be explored and stones removed. Similarly, if the gallbladder is acutely inflamed and contains stones, evacuation of stones from the gallbladder may also be accomplished and the gallbladder drained separately. Prolonged surgical procedures with deep anesthesia and blood loss are poorly tolerated by these extremely ill patients, and in the most severe types of the disease, surgery should be confined to the simplest drainage of the common duct and gallbladder. There is a great temptation for the surgeon to extend his attempts to improve the condition of these patients before surgery is undertaken. Conservative therapy, however, has been unsuccessful; so far there have been no survivors without surgical intervention.[59] Even with expeditious surgery, the mortality is high, between 35 and 50 per cent.[57-60] Preoperative preparation should be limited to the essentials, that is, rapid replacement of fluid losses along with concomitant intravenous administration of large doses of broad-spectrum antibiotics. Hypotension and shock may require the administration of steroids to support the patients.[60]

The cause of death in acute suppurative cholangitis is usually multiple liver abscesses, and although the superficial cause of death is often renal failure, the underlying cause is almost always the liver infection.

SCLEROSING CHOLANGITIS

Sclerosing cholangitis is a rather rare condition affecting males more often than females and occurring in all age groups, although it has not been described in infancy and is not necessarily related to cholelithiasis.[70] Scarring strictures and narrowing of the extra- and

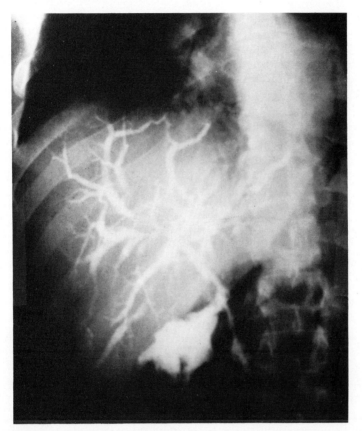

Figure 5–30 Sclerosing cholangitis. This operating room cholangiogram is from a 48 year old man with intermittent jaundice over a period of four years. The contrast material is injected through a needle in the hepatic duct. The segmental narrowing of branches of the intrahepatic ductal system is obvious. The hepatic and common ducts are almost completely obliterated distally, and the contrast material thus does not enter the duodenum. Grossly the bile duct was transformed into a hard, narrow, beaded cord of scar tissue. The patient was treated by a hepaticojejunostomy, Roux-Y type, without the use of steroids or long-term indwelling splints. He is well five years later.

intrahepatic bile ducts can be caused by many different entities from trauma to operative injury and infection.[64,67] In the case of biliary cirrhosis secondary to stones, narrowing of both the intra- and extrahepatic bile ducts may be seen; narrowing of the intrahepatic ducts may be caused by the primary cirrhosis alone, through distortion of the portal triads. Carcinoma of the bile ducts may cause narrowing over a considerable part of the biliary ductal system; this is the result of intramural spread of the cancer through the lymphatics in the walls of the ducts. Differentiation between the cancerous strictures of the bile ducts and the so-called benign sclerosing cholangitis is not always easy, since the cancer in this location may often be extremely slow-growing and histologically difficult to diagnose because of cirrhous growth, with the cancer cells only scattered in biopsy material.[69] Carcinomas of the bile ducts may remain localized and cause bile obstruction for such long periods of time that decompression by splinting tubes gives prolonged survival and thus may give the false impression that the surgeon has been dealing with a benign stricture rather than a cancerous growth.[68,69]

The diagnosis of primary sclerosing cholangitis is most often made by exclusion, but many criteria have been postulated that should be fulfilled before the diagnosis of so-called primary sclerosing cholangitis is made. It is generally accepted that calculi should not be found in the common duct or in the bile duct system, although they may be present in the gallbladder itself.[63,66] There should be no history of recent common duct operation or recent biliary tract operation. Cancer has to be ruled out by histological examination. Some authors feel that commonly associated diseases, such as ulcerative colitis, regional enteritis, and retroperitoneal fibrosis, should be excluded before the diagnosis of primary sclerosing cholangitis is made. When this restriction is added to the ones previously mentioned, the cases of true primary sclerosing cholangitis are few and far between.[70]

Symptoms

The symptoms and signs of sclerosing cholangitis cannot be distinguished from those of other diseases of the biliary tract without surgical exploration and biopsy. Most of these patients do complain of pain and indigestion similar to those found in patients with gallstones. They all have had jaundice, often intermittent and of the obstructive type. Even though jaundice may be absent, there are other signs of obstruction, such as elevated alkaline phosphatase levels and elevated serum cholesterol. Preoperative evaluation through intravenous cholangiography is rather unrewarding; usually there is failure of visualization of the ductal system, although at times the system may by visualized and look somewhat more narrowed than would be expected, thus giving a clue to the diagnosis.

Etiology

The most common causes of sclerosing cholangitis are bacteremia and infection, originating in the intestine[65] and carried by the portal venous system. This would explain the fairly common occurrence of sclerosing cholangitis in patients with diseases such as ulcerative colitis and regional enteritis. Some authors have speculated that auto-immune phenomenon might be responsible for the disease, but this is now considered unlikely since patients on both steroid drugs and immunosuppressant therapy have been observed to develop sclerosing cholangitis. Ulcerative colitis was found in 12 of 51 patients reported by Brantigan, and two others in the same series were found to have regional enteritis.[63]

Findings at Operation

The findings at operation in sclerosing cholangitis may vary considerably. The liver may appear normal, but there are also numerous cases on record in which frank cirrhosis was present. The gallbladder may be normal or thickened and fibrotic, and occasionally stones may be present. The common bile duct, when it is involved, is hard, perhaps somewhat nodular, and only occasionally enlarged. Lymph nodes are found in the porta hepatis or around the bile duct. When the lumen of the bile duct is opened, the wall is found to be thickened and fibrous. The lumen is narrowed and may appear obliterated at times. Cholangiograms reveal the involvement of the ductal system, which may be localized or extend throughout the extra- and intrahepatic ductal system. Microscopically, there is extensive fibrosis in the ductal wall, with a reasonably normal mucosal lining inside.

Surgery

The surgery of sclerosing cholangitis tries first to establish the diagnosis and second to decompress the ductal system to relieve the jaundice and provide drainage of the bile to the intestine. This has been accomplished by many different means, occasionally through cholecystostomy when the involvement of the ductal system was

distal to cystic duct anastomosis to the hepatic duct. Hepaticojejunostomy can be used when the extrahepatic ductal system is found to be
too narrow to provide decompression through the insertion of a
T-tube. Most of the patients reported have been decompressed
through an indwelling T-tube, usually of a small caliber. The tube is
left in for a prolonged period of time, and occasionally dilatation of
the ductal system may occur following the decompression. In time
the tube is removed and lasting improvement occurs. The use of
steroids or immunosuppressive therapy is debatable and is not to be
relied upon.[64] Patients on steroid therapy have been found to develop
cholangitis and liver abscess, and the reports of improvement on
steroid therapy are not impressive enough to warrant universal use.
When sclerosing cholangitis is clearly secondary to ulcerative colitis
or regional enteritis, there may be reasonable cause to use steroids
and anticipate results in line with improvement in the primary
disease.

BENIGN DISORDERS CAUSING STENOSIS OF THE
LOWER END OF THE COMMON BILE DUCT

The term "benign" is used advisedly, mainly to distinguish this
condition from the obstruction of the lower end of the common duct
caused by malignant tumors. Certainly the disease, benign though it
may be, that causes obstruction of the lower end of the common duct
is not innocuous to the patient, since almost without exception surgery is involved in its correction. The surgery involved is complicated
and entails considerable morbidity, and there is no general agreement
on which type of operation to use for any of these different problems.

The most common cause of stenosis in the lower end of the common duct is gallstones, located either in the gallbladder or in the
common duct. The infection and damage from stones cause fibrosis,
scarring, and contracture of the duct that ultimately result in obstruction, although it may take many years to develop to that point. The
strictures in the common duct are commonly of two types. One type
of stricture is short and limited to and located at the ampulla of Vater,
with an even dilatation of the bile duct from the ampulla of Vater up
into the liver. This is sometimes only a membranous stricture, with a
thin membrane of scarred ampulla causing the narrowing and imped-
iment to the bile flow. The second type of stricture is more extensive,
usually involves the intrapancreatic and intraduodenal portions of the
common duct, and is 2 or 3 cm in length. The dilatation of the duct
only becomes apparent at the upper border of the duodenum. This
stricture is commonly caused by stones residing in the lower end of
the common duct or by recurrent attacks of pancreatitis associated

with stones. This long stricture may also be caused by damage to the duct during surgical intervention. The damage probably most commonly occurs during gastric surgery in which difficult duodenal ulcers are being removed, and the duct is injured during surgery performed in inflammatory tissues. Chronic recurrent pancreatitis of nonbiliary origin, most commonly due to alcohol ingestion, may in its later stages cause stricture of the lower end of the common duct. Recurrent bouts of acute pancreatitis, alcoholic or otherwise, frequently cause obstructive jaundice during the acute attack. This jaundice is caused by the impingement of the inflammatory process from the surrounding pancreas on the common duct and usually resolves when the attack of pancreatitis subsides. When recurrent attacks of pancreatitis occur over a period of years, the scar formation in the pancreas and surrounding tissues may involve the periductal tissues, and the duct may become involved in the sclerosing process of the shrinking pancreatic tissues and thus become occluded. This stricture is long, since it involves the entire retroduodenal portion of the common duct. Another cause of strictures is perforation of the duct during exploration; damage may occur in the pancreatic tissues of the periduodenal area, causing postoperative abscesses and inflammation which may lead to permanent scar formation and narrowing of the duct. Occasionally, parts of instruments are broken off during common duct exploration and are left inside the duct or imbedded in the tissue around it, only to form an inflammatory mass that encroaches on and slowly occludes the duct through scar formation. Very uncommonly, large posterior duodenal ulcers may encroach on the common duct and cause mild jaundice and obstruction. Ordinarily, this jaundice disappears when the ulcer is treated, and the inflammatory reaction around the ulcer recedes and improves. Permanent stricture formation at the lower end of the common duct in duodenal ulcers is extremely rare, even when choledochoduodenal fistulas have occurred from penetration of the ulcer into the common bile duct.

Symptoms

The accurate diagnosis of the extent and type of strictures at the lower end of the common duct can only be made at the time of surgery, although intravenous cholangiography and transduodenal cannulation of the ampulla of Vater may aid considerably in appropriate cases. The symptoms of the obstructing lesions are nonspecific and are similar to many types of common duct obstruction whether from stones, pancreatitis, or even malignant tumors.

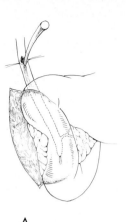

A

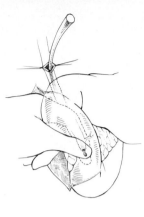

B

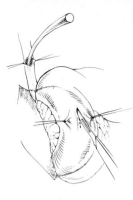

C

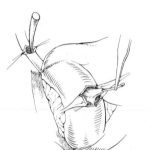

D

E

F

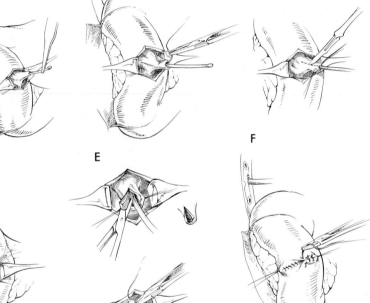

G

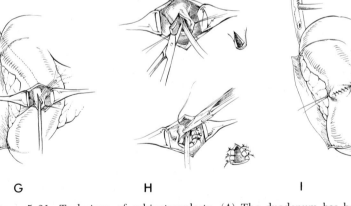

H

I

Figure 5–31   Technique of sphincteroplasty. (*A*) The duodenum has been rotated medially through the Kocher maneuver. A small choledochotomy has been done, and a flexible bougie has been passed through the ampulla of Vater. (*B*) Palpation of the bougie in the common bile duct allows determination of the location of the ampulla of Vater. (*C*) A very small duodenotomy is done between stay sutures opposite to the ampulla of Vater. (*D*) The bougie is pulled out of the duodenotomy. The ampulla is drawn tight over the bougie and stands out as a tight ring. (*E*) Sutures are placed around the sphincter of Oddi, and the needles are slid off the bougie. (*F*) A sphincterotomy is done with the bougie in place between the stay sutures. (*G*) A silver probe is placed

(*Continued on opposite page.*)

Sphincteroplasty and Duodenotomy for Stricture
and Impacted Stone

Sphincterotomy has been performed through the common bile duct and through the duodenum. In order for the procedure to be done safely and adequately, the surgeon must be able to visualize the ampulla of Vater and to control the bleeding that may ensue. Only the transduodenal approach fulfills these criteria and is now almost exclusively used.[71,74,76] The reasons for the use of sphincterotomy or sphincteroplasty are enumerated in various sections in the text, but the most common are stenosis of the sphincter with outflow obstruction in the common duct, an impacted stone that cannot be removed through the common bile duct, and the need to find and explore the pancreatic duct of Wirsung. Sphincteroplasty is an effective way of dealing with short or membranous strictures at the lower end of the common duct. Duodenotomy in biliary surgery is almost always performed to gain access to the sphincter of Oddi or ampulla of Vater. The reasons that lead to duodenotomy for dividing the sphincter and gaining access to the lowest part of the common bile duct are often difficulties in demonstrating patency of the lower end of the duct and its entrance into the duodenum. Failure to pass catheters, bougies, or other instruments into the duodenum during common duct exploration and failure of operative cholangiography to show patency of the duct are indications for duodenotomy and exploration of the sphincter of Oddi and ampulla from the duodenal side. A serious complication of duodenotomy is breakdown of the closure, with establishment of a side duodenal fistula and subsequent subhepatic abscess or peritonitis. The incidence and occurrence of duodenal fistulas are directly related to the ease with which the ampulla can be located. The location of the ampulla of Vater is not always certain, and it is not always easy to place the duodenotomy exactly opposite the ampulla. The ampulla itself may not be easily seen, although it usually can be palpated with the finger as a firm nubbin inside the duodenum. Visual inspection is hampered by the mucosal folds, and even after it is seen, it is difficult to get hold of it with forceps or sutures since the duodenal mucosa is friable. Once

---

Figure 5–31 (Continued)
into the pancreatic duct, which may be found in the lower right corner of the ampulla a few millimeters inside the ampullary ring. (*H*) With the probe in the pancreatic duct, a wedge of the ampulla of Vater attached to the outer stay suture is removed. The bile duct and duodenal mucosa are reapproximated, using interrupted sutures of 3 or 4–0 chromic catgut. The probe in the pancreatic duct prevents inclusion of the duct in the sutures. (*I*) The duodenotomy is closed transversely with interrupted sutures of fine silk. A short, thin T-tube is left in the common bile duct.

bleeding starts, identification becomes still more difficult. All too often the result is an ever enlarging duodenotomy, either by deliberate extension or by tearing due to retractors inserted for exposure. A large duodenotomy with traumatized edges thus sets the stage for insecure closure, an invitation to breakdown and fistula.

The problems of the difficult duodenotomy can be avoided when the location of the ampulla of Vater is known before the incision is made into the duodenum. Most of the time it is possible, with the common bile duct open, to pass a small-caliber bougie (filiform) past an obstructing stone or through a tight stricture. The bougie can be palpated through the duodenal wall where it emerges from the ampulla. A small duodenotomy is made over the ampulla, and the end of the bougie is pulled out of the duodenotomy; by lifting up the bougie, the ampulla of Vater is brought out of the duodenotomy with the sphincter of Oddi as a tight band encircling the bougie. Stay sutures can be placed around the sphincter by sliding the needle up along the bougie. The sphincter is then divided over the bougie between the stay sutures. The bougie can be delivered through the ampulla, usually bringing with it impacted stones.

The incision for the sphincterotomy should be done far away from the pancreatic duct. Since the pancreatic duct enters the ampulla medially and from behind, the sphincterotomy is made above and laterally. To be effective for gaining access to the ampulla of Vater, the sphincterotomy should be 2 cm long or longer. When the procedure is done for stenosis or stricture, a triangular wedge is removed from the circumference of the sphincter, and the duodenal mucosa and ampullary mucosa are approximated with interrupted catgut sutures on each side of the wedge. A probe should be placed in the pancreatic duct during suturing to prevent occlusion of the duct. At times, a probe cannot be passed into the duodenum. When this is the case, a fairly stiff bougie can still be placed as far distally as possible in the common bile duct. Palpation of the tip of this bougie through the duodenum gives approximate location of the ampulla, and with the duodenum open the bougie serves to lift the ampulla into view in the duodenotomy. In this instance, sutures must be placed in the sphincter without the aid of a splint, described earlier.

The common duct is drained with a T-tube following sphincterotomy. The T-tube used is short and does not go through to the duodenum across the sphincterotomy or the pancreatic duct. It is not considered necessary to use a long-arm T-tube for ensuring patency of the sphincteroplasty once a wedge has been removed from the sphincter and the edges reapproximated with sutures. It may also be damaging to the area of the sphincter and the pancreatic duct to have a tube going across it; on occasion, when the lower end is inside the duodenum, duodenal contents may be siphoned up through the tube,

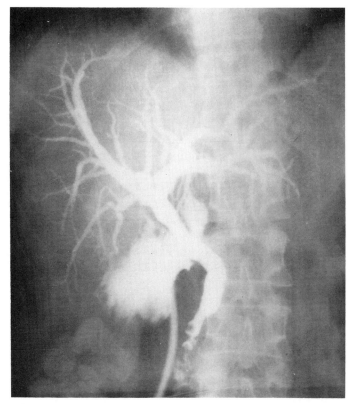

Figure 5-32 Common duct stones impacted in the lower end of the bile duct at and proximal to the ampulla of Vater. After common bile duct stones were removed, bougies and catheters could not be passed into the duodenum. A T-tube cholangiogram shows the calculi impacted in the lower end of the common bile duct. These stones could not be removed by the usual methods through a choledochotomy. A duodenotomy and sphincterotomy were performed, and the stones were removed easily through the lower end of the bile duct.

thus blocking bile drainage. The duodenotomy is closed in layers with interrupted sutures of fine silk.

The dangers of sphincterotomy and sphincteroplasty in the past have usually been related to postoperative pancreatitis or leakage from the site of the duodenotomy. Both these complications can be avoided to a great extent by gentle and thoughtful exploration of the ducts prior to sphincterotomy, using nonrigid instruments and as little force as possible in probing of the common duct and probing for the duodenum. I have found it inadvisable to use pointed metallic instruments for the above reasons. It is true that perforation of the common duct may occur from any instrument incorrectly used, but metallic probes of small caliber seem to invite trouble for those unwary and not thoroughly trained in their use. When a probe cannot be passed into the duodenum without excessive force, the ampulla can still be identified by a bougie in the lower end of the common duct that indents the posterior aspect of the duodenum in the region of the ampulla, as described earlier.

Choledochoduodenostomy and Choledochojejunostomy

Strictures that involve most of the retroduodenal portion of the common bile duct are not amenable to surgery through sphincterotomy or sphincteroplasty and are better treated either through choledochoduodenostomy[72,73,75,78] or choledochojejunostomy. Both operations are quite effective and give good results when properly used and correctly performed. This discussion does not concern the use of these procedures for recurrent stones or obstruction of the common bile duct due to stones alone, in which case removal of the stones would ordinarily be sufficient to take care of the obstruction. Rather, it deals with the use of these procedures when the obstruction to the bile flow is caused by an organic stricture in the wall of the duct.

Choledochoduodenostomy is a good procedure for stricture of this kind, but proper selection of the patients is important. Thus the patient selected for a choledochoduodenostomy has to have a dilated common duct and also a freely mobile duodenum, so that the duodenum and common duct can be approximated without any tension on the suture lines. The common duct used for choledochoduodenostomy should be at least 2.5 cm in diameter; in that situation, an anastomosis can best be accomplished through a transverse incision in the common duct as low down and as close to the duodenum as possible. The use of a vertical incision for a choledochoduodenostomy is not as advantageous, but the surgeon may be faced with having to use an incision of this kind if indications for the operation are not apparent until after a standard common duct exploration. It is advisable to bear the possibility in mind that, the closer to the duodenum the choledochotomy is, the less likely are difficulties to occur with anastomosis to the duodenum, should this become necessary. The choledochoduodenostomy should be done through a transverse incision in the common duct and through a parallel incision in the duodenum whenever possible. The posterior anastomosis is done with interrupted sutures of fine silk, then a second layer of chromic catgut. The anterior layer is similarly done after thorough mobilization of the duodenum through the Kocher maneuver, so that the duodenum can be displaced and rolled up on the common duct, taking any tension off the anastomosis. Usually the bile duct is decompressed after choledochoduodenostomy by a straight catheter which is placed through the cystic duct or the cystic duct stump and which does not cross the anastomotic line.

A choledochojejunostomy should be performed in those circumstances in which a common duct is not large enough or in which scarring, inflammation, or fixation prevents proper approximation of the duodenum and the common duct without tension.

Choledochojejunostomy for Distal Stricture of the Common Bile Duct

A choledochojejunostomy rather than a choledochoduodenostomy should be used in distal stricture when the size of the common duct is not large enough to provide an adequate size anastomosis, when scarring and fixation prevent adequate mobilization of the duodenum for this anastomosis, or when a stricture extends farther up the common bile duct than the duodenum will reach. The choledochojejunostomy is done using the Roux-Y principle. The first available loop of small bowel distal to the ligament of Treitz is selected, and the distal end of the divided bowel is brought either through the mesocolon or anterior to the colon up to the common bile duct. The anastomosis can be done either end-to-side or end-to-end. Depending on the circumstances, the duct can be divided and then implanted into the end of the jejunum, or the end of the jejunum can be anastomosed to a longitudinal incision on the anterior aspect of the bile duct. It is not essential to do an accurate mucosa-to-mucosa anastomosis; rather, a splinting catheter is placed up through the loop of jejunum into the hepatic duct, and the jejunum is anastomosed to the sides of the common bile duct around the incision or even to tissues in the porta hepatis. To prevent dislocation of the splinting catheter during the postoperative period, the catheter should be fixed to the jejunum with a suture of catgut (described in the repair of bile duct fistulas and strictures) and buried in the jejunum in a Witzel-type fashion. The procedure is completed by end-to-side anastomosis of the proximal jejunum to the ascending limb.

Both procedures have advantages. The choledochoduodenostomy empties the bile properly into the duodenum, where early and normal mixing with the food exiting from the stomach occurs. The choledochoduodenostomy is often a simpler, faster, and less time-consuming procedure, which is particularly important when dealing with elderly or debilitated patients. The disadvantage of a choledochoduodenostomy is the possibility that a side duodenal fistula will result when a breakdown of the anastomosis between the duct and the duodenum occurs. This is a combined biliary-pancreatic-duodenal fistula, which is often extremely difficult to heal with conservative measures and which entails a high morbidity and mortality. The choledochojejunostomy, on the other hand, takes more time to perform. It does not provide normal mixing of the bile with the food that leaves the stomach. It involves two anastomoses – one between the bowel and the biliary tree, and one between the two parts of the bowel itself. The advantages of the choledochojejunostomy are that risks of duodenal fistula are eliminated, and biliary fistulas are highly unlikely to occur. When they do occur, they are not nearly as serious as the combined biliary-pancreatic-duodenal fistula. The risk of postoperative cholangitis is probably the same for both procedures. It is my belief that cholangitis following choledochoduodenostomy is not based on reflux of gastric contents into the biliary tree but rather on narrowing and obstruction of the anastomosis between the biliary tree and the intestine. Moreover, the fever and sepsis are based on inability to evacuate the biliary tree rather than on passage of intestinal contents through the anastomosis. The same problem also applies to the choledochojejunostomy; cholangitis and jaundice are not seen here unless and until such time that the anastomosis has scarred and a stricture has formed, which prevents adequate emptying of the biliary tree into the intestinal loop.

Choledochoduodenostomy or Sphincteroplasty for Primary or Recurrent Common Duct Stones

The use of choledochoduodenostomy or sphincteroplasty has been recommended in patients with multiple stones in the common duct, with recurrent common bile duct stones, and with intrahepatic calculi, but it is still a controversial subject. The doubt surrounding the use of biliary intestinal anastomosis for the relief of primary or recurrent common duct stones requires some explanation.[77-79] The nature and cause of common duct stones are no more clear than the nature and cause of gallstones in general. It is reasonable to assume, however, that most common duct stones have their origin in the gallbladder and later reach their eventual size in the common bile duct. Although there are well-documented cases in which stones have been found in the common bile duct and not in the gallbladder and in which people with congenital absence of the gallbladder have been found to harbor common duct stones, these exceptions are so rare that, for all practical purposes, we have to assume that the origin of most common duct stones is in the gallbladder itself. The incidence of common duct stones following cholecystectomy – that is, discovered in a patient who has already had a previous cholecystectomy and perhaps a common duct exploration – is between 4 and 6 per cent, whereas about 12 per cent of the patients who are admitted to the hospital for gallbladder stones are found to have common duct stones.

Among the 4 to 6 per cent of patients who have recurrent common duct stones, there is a further small number in whom stone formation seems to be continuous and to proceed irrespective of how often calculi are removed from the biliary tree. It is fairly obvious that, for this small number of people with recurrent common duct stones, simple removal from the biliary tree is not sufficient, and the problem is to find a way to prevent formation of the stones, to facilitate their passage, or to bypass potential obstruction. A certain number of these patients with recurrent stone formation have a dilated common bile duct with a narrowing at its distal end; perhaps stasis and infection in the biliary tree proximal to an area of stenosis predispose to the formation of the stones. It is not unreasonable that, in this instance, an attempt should be made to relieve the obstruction in the biliary tree at the same time that the stones are removed. The obstruction found in association with the dilated common bile duct containing stones can be of many types. One type is the formation of a fine scar with stenosis of the ampulla, as described previously, for which sphincteroplasty is indicated. For other patients with an established long stricture and recurrent common duct stones not amenable to sphincteroplasty, biliary intestinal anastomosis is indicated, following the same lines of reasoning and methods as already described using either choledochoduodenostomy or choledochojejunostomy.

Other patients do not seem to have a truly established stricture but rather a narrower caliber, or perhaps a normal caliber, of the duct at the ampulla of Vater that is easily dilated with bougies and seems to retain its normal pliability. The problem arises here of what to do for these patients who do not have a true organic stricture in the bile duct but still have a dilated bile duct with recurrent stone formation. Adequate drainage of the duct to eliminate stasis can be accomplished in some of these people, but rarely with a sphincteroplasty. Sphincteroplasty will, in selected instances, afford good emptying of the dilated duct and thus prevent stone formation by providing dependent drainage. An alternate choice is to divide the duct and do an end-to-end choledochojejunostomy, which will give dependent drainage and may also pass reformed stones into the intestine. The chances of stenosis with choledochojejunostomy are probably somewhat less than those with a well done sphincteroplasty. A choledochoduodenostomy in this instance drains the common bile duct at a level higher than its most dependent portion, that is, the ampulla of Vater. It therefore provides drainage of bile without eliminating the stasis in its lower portion. As long as there is an anastomosis that remains open, attacks of frank cholangitis are no more likely to occur than with other types of anastomosis, and numerous surgeons can quote a series of patients in whom they claim this operation has been used with excellent results. There is, however, a blind pouch distal to the anastomosis, and reformed stones are likely to collect in this pouch and later cause symptoms, although obstructive jaundice is usually avoided.

All these procedures for recurrent common duct stones are applicable and useful on rare occasions in the patients who are habitual stone-formers, or when the surgeon finds it impossible to remove all the concretions, which is particularly apt to happen with intra-hepatic stones. It should be remembered, however, that these procedures are a second line of defense and should not be used instead of a thorough bile duct exploration with stone removal, which, when properly performed, is so effective in most patients.

BILIARY ENTERIC FISTULAS

Biliary enteric fistulas are rare, being found in only about 0.2 to 1 per cent of biliary tract operations.[80] They are caused by stones eroding through the walls of the biliary tract and entering an adjacent hollow viscus or rarely by the erosion of a carcinomatous growth in the biliary tree or the intestine into the adjacent organ.[81,82,85,96] Also rare but still occasionally seen are biliary enteric fistulas caused by benign peptic ulcers of the duodenum or the stomach that penetrate into the common bile duct rather than the gallbladder.[83,89,94] Fistulas from trauma are also seen.[90] The most common cause of biliary enteric fistulas is the presence of stones in the biliary tree that erode into the duodenum, stomach, or colon.[90]

The history of the fistula ordinarily includes a long-standing, chronic cholecystitis and cholelithiasis with intermittent attacks of acute obstructive cholecystitis. When attacks of acute cholecystitis occur, the gallbladder is walled off from the rest of the abdominal cavity by the adjacent organs—the duodenum, the lower end of the stomach, and the transverse colon. When perforation and penetration of the gallbladder wall due to gangrene occur, the stones in the gall-bladder rest immediately on the wall of the adjacent organ and slowly burrow through by pressure necrosis, establishing the fistula. Most commonly the fistula is between the body of the gallbladder and the duodenum, but the ampulla is also frequently the site of the fistula formation. Much more rarely the fistula leads into the transverse colon (in which case profuse diarrhea often develops)[87,91] or into the pylorus or the antrum of the stomach.[97] Many biliary enteric fistulas are insidious and do not cause any signs or symptoms beyond those seen in recurrent attacks of cholecystitis. Thus many of these fistulas are discovered only accidentally during cholecystectomy for chronic biliary disease.[92] Much more rare are fistulas between the common duct and intestine. These do occur but are seen much more rarely now since elective biliary tract surgery has become easily available. Biliary enteric fistulas were commonly found prior to the development of modern biliary tract surgery. It is understandable that the largest series collected on biliary enteric fistulas was done by Courvoisier in 1890. In Courvoisier's day and before, biliary enteric fistulas were often the only means by which patients recovered from obstruction of the biliary passages due to gallstones.

Incidence

Biliary enteric fistulas from gallstones are becoming more and more rare as elective surgery becomes more accepted. They occur more often in women than in men, in direct relation to the more commen occurrence of gallstones in women. It is a disease of middle and old age, and although it may be seen in patients in their thirties and

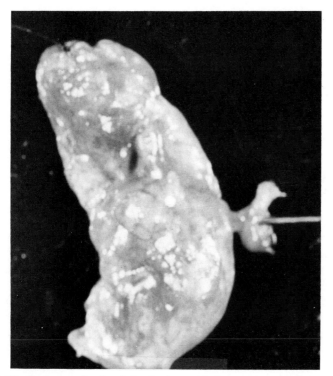

Figure 5–33 Cholecystoduodenal fistula. Many cholecystoenteric fistulas are found incidentally during elective surgery for gallstones. This fistula was between the duodenum and the midportion of the gallbladder. The fistula was easily dismantled by excising a small portion of the duodenal wall, which was then closed. The probe extends through the fistulous tract from the duodenal site into the gallbladder.

younger, it is most commonly seen in the fifth and sixth decades and has been encountered in people in the ninth decade. This complication of biliary tract disease is rather rare, and a biliary enteric fistula is encountered about once in every 100 operations for gallstones.

Symptoms and Signs

As mentioned earlier, the symptoms and signs of biliary enteric fistulas are few and are often indistinguishable from the classic symptoms of cholecystitis and cholelithiasis. When symptoms are nonspecific, the fistula is usually found accidentally at operation. Frequently the patients give a long history of gallbladder problems, but there are exceptions to this also. The classic findings in biliary enteric fistulas are seen when they are associated with gallstone ileus or obstruction.[86,88,92] Once the fistula has been established, the stones harbored in the gallbladder are extruded into the intestinal tract and undoubtedly sometimes passed through the rectum without causing significant problems. However, at times obstruction occurs, and the incidence of obstruction is directly related to the size of the stone extruded into the intestine. When the fistula forms between the gallbladder and the pylorus of the stomach, which happens rarely, the pyloric obstruction is usually early and significant. A much more common site of fistulas is between the gallbladder and duodenum, where most biliary intestinal fistulas join the intestinal tract. The stones passed into the duodenum move down the small intestine and, if they are of sufficient size, cause obstruction in the terminal ileum or sometimes higher up in the jejunum. Gallstones passed from the gallbladder into the transverse colon usually cause large bowel obstruction, specifically in the sigmoid colon.

Patients with strictures or narrowing of the intestinal tract from previous inflammatory diseases, such as diverticulitis or intestinal surgery, are more likely to develop obstruction from gallstones, and smaller stones cause obstruction in these patients than in those without preexisting disease in the intestines. Thus the patient with gallstone ileus is usually a woman who has had known gallstones or symptoms of biliary tract disease for a long period of time with intermittent attacks of cholecystitis. Commonly there is a history of or evidence of jaundice immediately preceding the onset of the obstruction, which is then followed by the crampy abdominal pain, nausea, and vomiting typical of small bowel obstruction.

X-rays of the abdomen may be diagnostic. There is air seen in the biliary tree as evidence of communication between the biliary tree and the intestine. There is evidence of small bowel obstruction or, more rarely, of gastric obstruction or large bowel obstruction, and on occasion the large calcified gallstone may be seen within the intestine. It is quite rare, however, that all the classic findings of gallstone ileus are present.

Biliary Enteric Fistulas Caused by Peptic Ulcer

The biliary enteric fistulas caused by peptic ulcer constitute a special group. These do not lead to, and are not associated with, gall-stone ileus and are rarely associated with gallstones at all. Usually the fistulas extend from the duodenum[83,91,94] to the common bile duct, but rarely gastric ulcers may penetrate the biliary tree.[97] Biliary fistulas from ulcers rarely cause symptoms from the biliary tree;[83] rather, the symptoms are from the ulcer, and the fistula is only found accidentally on barium x-rays by reflux into the biliary tree or by the finding of air in the biliary tree on scout films of the abdomen. The treatment in these situations is usually aimed at the ulcer, and the biliary fistula is ignored. When the common duct is patent beyond the fistula, it will usually close with healing of the ulcer. A simple gastroenterostomy and vagectomy may thus be the treatment of choice in the case of a duodenal ulcer with a fistula. Occasionally the peptic ulcer needs to be removed because of profuse bleeding.[94] In such instances the duodenal stump is sutured around the fistula to allow drainage. Common bile duct fistula with ulcer and scarring and obliteration of the distal bile duct have been reported. Whenever the fistula is compromised during the operation for ulcer, it is incumbent upon the surgeon to demonstrate patency of the bile duct beyond the fistula. Establishment of common bile duct drainage by T-tube is also advisable to avoid biliary leak into the abdomen postoperatively.

Gallstone Ileus

Gallstones are an uncommon cause of intestinal obstruction. They usually have to be large, over 2.5 cm in diameter, to cause obstruction, although smaller stones can cause obstruction when organic narrow-ing of the intestine is present, such as strictures or neoplasm. Not more than 1 to 3 per cent of intestinal obstruction is caused by gall-stones.[84] On the other hand, when only the older patients are consid-ered, gallstones may be the cause of obstruction in up to 24 per cent of patients over the age of 70.[84] The patients with gallstone ileus are rarely diagnosed preoperatively; in no more than one out of three is the correct diagnosis established prior to surgery.[86] Thus the surgeon is usually faced with patients with small or large bowel obstruction of unknown etiology. Up to this point intestinal obstruction is treated according to the need established in each case. Occasionally the obstruction from the gallstone is intermittent, apparently based on the stone moving back and forth. In this case contrast studies can be performed and possibly the correct diagnosis established through use of the barium enema or the upper gastrointestinal examination.[92, 95] The presence of unrelieved small bowel or large bowel obstruction, however, usually indicates early surgery, and operation is begun following proper preparation of the patient by replacing fluid and electrolyte losses and correcting any obvious infirmities of other vital systems. The diagnosis is established during surgery when the obstructing gallstone is palpated in the small or large intestine. It is important to realize that more than one stone may be present, and the small and large intestines should be examined carefully for the presence of other calculi.

Relief of the obstruction depends on the location of the calculus. In the small bowel, the most common site is the terminal ileum, and the most commonly employed procedure is to move the stone proximally into the dilated part of the small bowel and in this area to do an enterotomy and remove the calculus. Prior to enterotomy, the intestine is occluded on both sides of the stone to prevent any spillage of intestinal contents at the time of removal. In the large bowel, the obstruction is commonly in the sigmoid and quite often associated with or caused by organic narrowing of the sigmoid colon from preexisting inflammatory disease, such as diverticulitis. The choice of operation here becomes more complicated. On rare occasions, a stone may be pushed through the narrowed area down into the rectum and the obstruction thus relieved without opening the intestine. More often, the stone can only be moved proximally into the dilated and obstructed part of the colon and there removed through enterotomy, as it is in the small bowel. At times the stone is imbedded in an inflammatory mass in the sigmoid colon, and it may be difficult to establish whether the calculus is the sole cause of the obstruction. In these instances and when closure of a colotomy seems to be precarious, establishment of a transverse colostomy is indicated. In exceptional circumstances, a calculus causing small bowel obstruction is impacted. This is more likely when an organic narrowing of the small bowel is present at the site of obstruction. It may then be impossible to dislodge the calculus from the area in the small bowel. If it can be dislodged, the intestine is often found so damaged that its viability is in question. In these instances a resection of the intestine should be undertaken. This should be done rather than a simple bypass procedure, since the calculus will undoubtedly erode through the intestinal wall in time and cause further problems.

Once a gallstone has been demonstrated as the cause of intestinal obstruction, the surgeon immediately knows that disease is also present in the biliary tree. Exploration and palpation of the gallbladder area at this time will often establish the presence of an inflammatory mass or an inflamed gallbladder, possibly still containing calculi. The surgeon then has to choose whether to proceed with correction of the biliary tract disease or whether to be satisfied with correction of the intestinal obstruction and plan his biliary tract procedure for a later time. The choice here is simple if the patient involved is seriously ill from the intestinal obstruction or is in precarious health from other ailments. The wisest course then undoubtedly is to be satisfied with correction of the intestinal obstruction. If on the other hand, the patient is reasonably young and in good health, the obstruction is of recent onset, and the examination of the gallbladder reveals minimal or moderate inflammatory reaction rather than a large inflammatory mass, it is permissible to proceed with cholecystectomy and closure of the fistula at the same time as the intestinal obstruction is relieved. However, these patients should represent the exception rather than the rule. An exception may exist when the patient, in addition to the intestinal obstruction, has obstructive jaundice. Obstructive jaundice does require surgical correction at the earliest possible opportunity, and a surgeon may be forced into a simple drainage of the bile duct at the time of the initial surgery. The reason for delaying biliary tract surgery in old, debilitated, and critically ill patients is the fact that the biliary intestinal fistulas in the early stages are often quite large. Thus closure of the duodenum following cholecystectomy can be problematic because of the size of the defect in the duodenal wall. Similarly, simple drainage of the gallbladder at the time of operation for the intestinal obstruction could be ill-advised, since this may establish a duodenal fistula through the gallbladder. Finally, the incidence of common duct stones is high in patients with biliary enteric fistulas, and a common duct exploration should be a routine part of correction of the biliary disease. All these procedures are better done later during a planned elective operation unless the condition of the patient is such that the biliary tract disease could be immediately life-threatening. Mortality from surgery for gallstone ileus is now reported between 13 and 15 per cent.[81,84]

REFERENCES

1. Abu Dahn, J., and Chica, J.: Acute cholecystitis with perforation into the peritoneal cavity. Arch. Surg. 102:108, 1971.
2. Bockus, H. L.: Gastroenterology. 2nd ed. Vol. III. Philadelphia, W. B. Saunders Company, 1963.
3. Cafferata, H. T., Stallone, R. J., and Mattewson, C. W.: Acute cholecystitis in a municipal hospital: The role and results of cholecystostomy. Arch. Surg. 98:435, 1969.

4. Chang, F. C.: Intravenous cholangiography in the diagnosis of acute cholecystitis. Am. J. Surg. *120*:567, 1970.
5. Corlette, M. B., and Bismuth, H.: Acute cholecystitis and jaundice. Arch. Surg. *106*:829, 1973.
6. Fleming, R., et al.: Bacteriologic studies of biliary tract infection. Ann. Surg. *166*:563, 1967.
7. Gardner, B., et al.: Factors influencing the timing of cholecystectomy in acute cholecystitis. Am. J. Surg. *125*:730, 1973.
8. Glenn, F., and Wantz, G.: Acute cholecystitis following surgical treatment of unrelated disease. Surg. Gynecol. Obstet. *102*:145, 1956.
9. Glenn, F., and Thorbjarnarson, B.: The surgical treatment of acute cholecystitis. Surg. Gynecol. Obstet. *116*:61, 1963.
10. Hauman, R. L., and Anderson, M. C.: Effect of specific pancreatic enzymes on the gallbladder. Surg. Forum *21*:388, 1970.
11. Laws, H. L., and Elliott, R. L.: Postoperative acalculous gangrenous cholecystitis. Ann. Surg. *37*:371, 1971.
12. Lindberg, E. F., et al.: Acalculous cholecystitis in Vietnam casualties. Ann. Surg. *171*:152, 1970.
13. McCubbrey, D., and Thieme, T.: In defense of the conservative treatment for acute cholecystitis with an evaluation of the risk involved. Surgery *45*:930, 1959.
14. Munster, A. M., and Brown, J. R.: Acalculous cholecystitis. Am. J. Surg. *113*:730, 1967.
15. Rosenberg, S. A., and Buchanan, J. J.: Acute acalculous cholecystitis unrelated to previous operation. Ann. Surg. *32*:319, 1966.
16. Shaw, P. C.: Post-traumatic acute acalculous cholecystitis in young males. Milit. Med. *135*:210, 1970.
17. Strode, J. E.: Acute cholecystitis, an unexpected complication following surgery. Surg. Clin. North Am. *50*:357, 1970.
18. Thorbjarnarson, B.: Carcinoma of the gallbladder and acute cholecystitis. Ann. Surg. *151*:241, 1960.
19. Thorpe, C. D., Olsen, W. R., Fischer, H., Doust, V. L., and Joseph, R. R.: Emergency intravenous cholangiography in patients with acute abdominal pain. Am. J. Surg. *46*:50, 1973.
20. Watkin, D. F. L., and Thomas, G. G.: Jaundice in acute cholecystitis. Br. J. Surg. *58*:570, 1971.
21. Welder, R. S., et al.: Acute noncalculous cholecystitis axxociated with severe injury. Am. J. Surg. *119*:729, 1970.
22. Cholecystectomy in Ohio: Result of surgery in Ohio hospitals. Am. J. Surg. *119*:714, 1970.
23. Alexander, S., and McAlpine, F. S.: Cholecystectomy in the cardiac patient. Med. Clin. North Am. *50*:495, 1966.
24. Finley, M.: Perforation of the gallbladder. Review of Surgery Sept., Oct., 1972, p. 377.
25. Gingrich, R. A., Awe, W. C., Boyden, A. M., and Peterson, C. G.: Cholecystostomy in acute cholecystitis. Am. J. Surg. *116*:310, 1968.
26. Ibach, J. R., Hume, H. A., and Erb, W. H.: Cholecystectomy in the aged. Surg. Gynecol. Obstet. *126*:523, 1968.
27. Sparkman, R. S.: Planned cholecystostomy. Am. Surg. *149*:746, 1959.
28. Holgersen, L. O., White, I. I., and West, J. P.: Emphysematous cholecystitis. Surgery *69*:102, 1971.
29. Hooelius, L.: Pneumo-cholecystitis. Acta Chir. Scand. *139*:410, 1973.
30. Rosoff, L., and Meyers, H.: Acute emphysematous cholecystitis. Am. J. Surg. *111*:410, 1966.
31. Sarmiento, R. V.: Emphysematous cholecystitis. Arch. Surg. *93*:1009, 1966.
32. Boyd, W.: Pathology for the Surgeon. 7th ed. Philadelphia, W. B. Saunders Company, 1956, p. 247.
33. Bricker, D. L., and Halper, B.: Adenomyoma of the gallbladder. Surgery *53*:615, 1963.
34. Dawson, J. L.: Cholecystitis and cholecystectomy. Clinics in Gastroenterology *2*:91, 1973.

35. Baker, J. O., et al.: Removal of a retained biliary stone without reoperation. Arch. Surg. 104:702, 1972.
36. Bartlett, M. K., and Waddell, W. R.: Indications for common duct exploration. New Engl. J. Med. 258:164, 1958.
37. Chafaney, C. J.: Removal of retained bile duct calculus without operation. Br. J. Surg. 56:312, 1969.
38. Colcock, B. P., and Liddle, H. V.: Common bile duct stones. New Engl. J. Med. 258:264, 1958.
39. Edward, R., Rucker, C., and Finby, N.: Intravenous cholangiography. Arch. Surg. 90:73, 1965.
40. Gardner, B.: Experiences with the use of intracholedochal heparinized saline for the treatment of retained common duct stones. Ann. Surg. 177:240, 1972.
41. Glenn, F.: Choledochotomy in nonmalignant disease of the biliary tract. Surg. Gynecol. Obstet. 124:974, 1967.
42. Flenn, F., and Beil, A. R.: Choledocholithiasis demonstrated at 586 operations. Surg. Gynecol. Obstet. 118:499, 1964.
43. Hall, R. C., Sakiyalak, P., Kim, S. K., Rogers, L. S., and Webb, W. R.: Failure of operative cholangiography to prevent relieved common duct stones. Am. J. Surg. 125:51, 1973.
44. Henzel, J. H., and DeWeese, M. S.: Common duct exploration with and without balloon-tipped biliary catheters. Arch. Surg. 103:199, 1971.
45. Hilton, H. D., and Griffin, W. T.: Common duct exploration in acute cholecystitis: Review of 100 consecutive cases. Surgery 65:269, 1969.
46. Jolly, P. C., Baker, J. W., Schmidt, H. M., Walker, J. H., and Holm, J. C.: Operative cholangiography: A case for its routine use. Ann. Surg. 168:551, 1968.
47. Knight, C. D.: Use of balloon-tipped catheter in exploration of the common duct. Am. J. Surg. 113:717, 1967.
48. Lipton, S., and Caralps-Riera, E. J.: The plasma clot extraction of biliary duct calculi. Surgery 70:746, 1971.
49. Magee, R. B., and MacDuffee, R. C.: One thousand consecutive cholecystectomies. Arch. Surg. 96:858, 1968.
50. Mahour, G. H., Wakim, K. C., and Ferris, D. O.: The common bile duct in man, its diameter and circumference. Ann. Surg. 165:415, 1967.
51. Mazzariello, R.: Removal of residual biliary tract calculi without reoperation. Surgery 67:566, 1970.
52. Patterson, H. C., Grice, O. D., and Bream, C. A.: Overlooked gallstones and their retrieval. Am. J. Surg. 125:257, 1973.
53. Shore, J. M., and Berci, G.: Operative management of calculi in the hepatic ducts. Am. J. Surg. 119:625, 1970.
54. Shore, J. M., and Shore, E.: Operative biliary endoscopy: Experience with the flexible choledochoscope in 100 consecutive choledocholithotomies. Ann. Surg. 171:269, 1970.
55. Wen, C. C., and Lee, H. C.: Intrahepatic stones. Ann. Surg. 175:166, 1972.
56. White, T. T., Waisman, H., Hopton, D., and Kavle, H.: Radiomanometry, flow rates, and cholangiography in the evaluation of common bile duct disease. A study of 220 cases. Am. J. Surg. 123:73, 1972.
57. Dow, R. W., and Lindenauer, S. M.: Acute obstructive cholangitis. Ann. Surg. 169:272, 1969.
58. Glenn, F., and Moody, F. G.: Acute obstructive suppurative cholangitis. Surg. Gynecol. Obstet. 113:265, 1961.
59. Haupert, A. P., Carey, L. C., Evans, W. E., and Ellison, E. H.: Acute suppurative cholangitis. Arch. Surg. 94:460, 1967.
60. Hinchly, E. T., and Couper, C. E.: Acute obstructive cholangitis. Am. J. Surg. 117:62, 1969.
61. Huang, T., Bass, J. A., and Williams, R. D.: The significance of biliary pressure in cholangitis. Arch. Surg. 98:629, 1969.
62. Reynolds, B. M., and Dougan, E. L.: Acute obstructive cholangitis. Ann. Surg. 150:299, 1952.
63. Brantigan, C. O., and Brantigan, O. C.: Primary sclerosing cholangitis. Am. Surg. 39:191, 1973.

64. Cutler, B., and Donaldson, G. A.: Primary sclerosing cholangitis and obliterative cholangitis. Am. J. Surg. *117*:502, 1969.
65. Eade, M. N., Cooke, T. W., and Brooke, B. N.: Liver disease in ulcerative colitis. II. The long term effect of colectomy. Ann. Intern. Med. 72:489, 1970.
66. Glenn, F., and Whitsell, J. C.: Primary sclerosing cholangitis. Surg. Gynecol. Obstet. *123*:1037, 1966.
67. Smith, M. P., and Loe, R. H.: Sclerosing cholangitis. Am. J. Surg. *110*:239, 1965.
68. Thorbjarnarson, B.: Carcinoma of the bile ducts. Cancer *12*:708, 1959.
69. Thorbjarnarson, B.: Carcinoma of the intrahepatic bile ducts. Arch. Surg. 77:908, 1958.
70. Whelton, M. J.: Sclerosing cholangitis. *In* Clinics in Gastroenterology, Vol. 2. Philadelphia, W. B. Saunders Company, 1973, p. 163.
71. Beattie, W. G., and Kuppusami, M.: Sphincteroplasty, an individualized operation: An anatomic study in autopsy material. Can. J. Surg. *15*:384, 1972.
72. Degenshein, G. A., and Hurwitz, A.: The techniques of side to side choledocho-duodenostomy. Surgery *61*:972, 1967.
73. Johnson, A. G., and Harding Rains, A. J.: Choledochoduodenostomy: A reappraisal of its indications based on a study of 64 patients. Br. J. Surg. 59:277, 1972.
74. Jones, S. A., and Smith, L. L.: A reappraisal of sphincteroplasty (not sphincter-otomy). Surgery *71*:565, 1972.
75. Madden, J. L., Chun, J. Y., Kandalaft, S., and Parekh, M.: Choledochoduoden-ostomy: An unjustly maligned surgical procedure. Am. J. Surg. *119*:45, 1970.
76. Reynolds, B. M., and Balsano, N. A.: A new method for sphincterotomy. Surg. Gynecol. Obstet. *132*:297, 1971.
77. Sawyer, R. B., and Sawyer, K. C.: Choledochoduodenostomy for gallstones. Arch. Surg. *102*:308, 1971.
78. Stuart, M., and Hoerr, S. O.: Late results of side to side choledochoduodenostomy and of transduodenal sphincterotomy for benign disorders. Am. J. Surg. *123*:67, 1972.
79. Thomas, C. G., Jr., Nicholoson, C. P., and Owen, J.: Effectiveness of choledocho-duodenostomy and transduodenal sphincterotomy in the treatment of benign obstruction of the common duct. Ann. Surg. *173*:845, 1971.
80. Amory, R. A., and Barker, H. O.: Multiple biliary enteric fistulas. Am. J. Surg. *111*:180, 1966.
81. Buetow, G. W., and Crampton, R. S.: Gallstone ileus. Arch. Surg. 86:504, 1963.
82. Clairidge, M.: Recurrent gallstone ileus. Br. J. Surg. *49*:134, 1961.
83. Constant, E., and Turcotte, J. G.: Choledochoduodenal fistula; complication of ulcer disease. Ann. Surg. *167*:220, 1968.
84. Cooperman, A. M., et al.: Changing concepts in the surgical treatment of gallstone ileus. Ann. Surg. *167*:377, 1968.
85. Dove, H. J., and Gould, L. V.: Gallstone ileus. Br. J. Surg. *49*:660, 1962.
86. Glenn, F., and Mannix, H.: Biliary enteric fistulas. Surg. Gynecol. Obstet. *105*:693, 1957.
87. Gudas, P. P.: Cholecysto-colonic fistula. Arch. Surg. 95:228, 1967.
88. Hudspeth, A. S., and McQuirt, W. F.: Gallstone ileus. Arch. Surg. *100*:668, 1970.
89. Isaacson, S., Appleby, L. N., and Hamilton, E.: Choledochoduodenal fistula due to peptic ulcer. J.A.M.A. *174*:2204, 1960.
90. McLeod, J. A.: Biliary tract fistula. Am. Surgeon 25:177, 1959.
91. Newhauser, G. M., and Thompson, J. C.: Cholecysto-duodeno-coli fistula. Ann. Surg. *163*:81, 1966.
92. Shehad, W. H.: Roentgenologic observations in cases of fistulas of the biliary tree. J.A.M.A. *174*:2204, 1960.
93. Tuell, S. W.: Gallstone ileus. Am. Surgeon *31*:473, 1965.
94. Wagner, G. R., and Passaro, E.: Choledochoduodenal fistula due to ulcer. Arch. Surg. *103*:21, 1971.
95. Whitcomb, J. G., Bromme, D. A., and Lovelace, W. R.: Barium enema reduction of gallstone ileus. Am. J. Surg. *106*:592, 1963.
96. Whitsell, F. B., Jr.: Gallstone ileus. Ann. Surg. 36:317, 1970.
97. Williams, G. D., and Hara, M.: Spontaneous choledochogastric fistula. Am. J. Surg. *112*:102, 1966.

Chapter Six

BILE DUCT INJURIES

We do not know with any degree of accuracy how frequently bile duct injuries occur during operations. They may occur as often as once in every 200 to 300 cholecystectomies and are seen often enough and are serious enough to warrant giving highest attention to their prevention and repair. The operation most commonly associated with bile duct injury is cholecystectomy; gastrectomy is the next most common. Injury to the bile duct is rarely seen following common bile duct exploration, but it may occur.

CAUSE OF INJURY

The reason for the bile duct injury is usually unknown. Known causes are unplanned maneuvers to stop major bleeding, in which hemostats may be placed across, or ligatures placed including, the ducts. Another well known cause is the performance of a cholecystectomy when inflammation is great, exposure is poor, and the gallbladder is intimately adherent to the hepatic duct. In this situation stones from the cystic duct or ampulla of the gallbladder may erode into the hepatic duct and encourage transection of the duct at that level. A third and perhaps the most common cause for bile duct injury is the gallbladder with a very short or absent cystic duct. When the ampulla is lifted out of the field, the common bile duct is stretched and simulates a cystic duct, which may be divided unless proper precautions are observed.

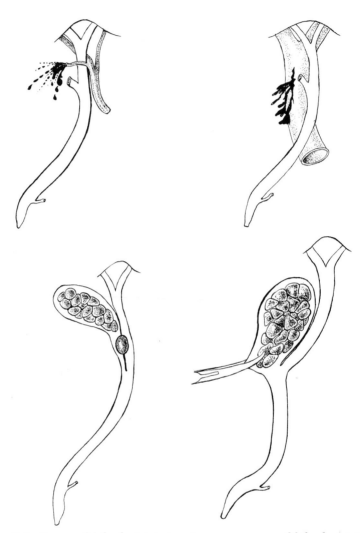

Figure 6–1 Causes of bile duct injuries. A common cause of bile duct injuries is massive, poorly controlled hemorrhage. The two upper drawings show bleeding from a cystic artery and from a portal vein. Unless such bleeding is first controlled by finger pressure on the hepatoduodenal ligament, there is danger of involving the bile duct with clamps or ligatures employed for hemostasis. The lower left hand picture shows a calculus in the cystic duct eroded into the common duct. This situation easily leads to confusion on the part of the operator, which results in transection of the hepatic duct at the level of the calculus. The lower right hand picture shows the gallbladder with very short or absent cystic duct. Traction on the ampulla of this gallbladder easily brings a small common duct into view and makes this appear to be the cystic duct. Unless care is exercised, the duct is divided at this point or ligated or both.

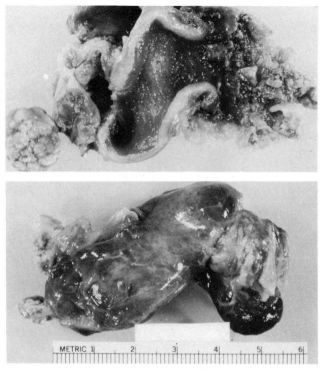

Figure 6–2 Bile duct injury. The specimen is a gallbladder with an attached segment of common bile duct. The segment of common bile duct is best seen in the lower photograph on the right side. The upper photograph shows a calculus in the lower left corner. This calculus had eroded from the cystic duct onto the common bile duct, leading to the transection and removal of the segment of common duct.

DIAGNOSIS

The patient with bile duct injury that is not detected at the time of surgery presents with either a biliary fistula or obstructive jaundice or both. Any patient who develops obstructive jaundice immediately following gallbladder operation or who drains large amounts of bile for over a week after a cholecystectomy should be considered to have a bile duct injury until it is proved otherwise.

Percutaneous cholangiography is indispensable as a diagnostic and preoperative measure in patients with obstructive jaundice, since this will accurately identify the level of the bile duct injury and clarify whether only the main bile duct or whether one or both hepatic ducts are involved. In the patient with biliary fistula, the site of injury can only rarely be identified preoperatively. Cannulation of the ampulla of Vater with retrograde cholangiography is possible in

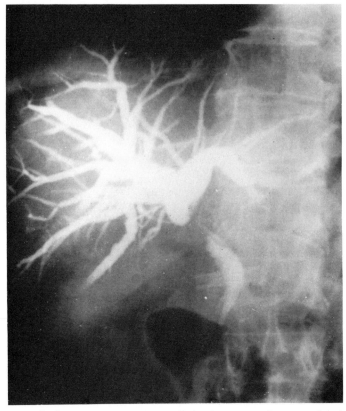

Figure 6–3   Bile duct injury in a patient with obstructive jaundice immediately follow-ing cholecystectomy. There was massive bleeding during a difficult cholecystectomy, and suture ligatures had to be employed to control the bleeding. Immediately post-operatively the patient became jaundiced. The percutaneous cholangiogram shown here was done three weeks following surgery. The cholangiogram shows a dilated intrahepatic ductal system and an obstruction low in the hepatic duct. Some contrast material entered the distal common duct but not enough to enter the duodenum. There is an obvious gap between the hepatic duct and the distal bile duct. At the time of surgery catgut ligatures were found around the lower end of the common hepatic duct. These ligatures were removed, a choledochotomy was done below the ligatures, and the duct was dilated in the area of the ligatures. The mucosa appeared intact, and a splinting T-tube was left in place for two months and then removed.

these patients, but it does not identify the proximal level of damage to the bile duct and thus is of limited value to the surgeon. Rarely, the bile duct may be identified on intravenous cholangiography and ex-travasation of the bile demonstrated. More often, success may be obtained by inserting catheters into the draining sinus and injecting dye. Both these methods for diagnosing the site of biliary fistula are inadequate and often unsuccessful, and therefore the diagnosis is usually only made at the time of exploratory surgery.

IMMEDIATE REPAIR OF BILE DUCT INJURY

The best time to perform a satisfactory repair of a bile duct injury is at the time of the primary operation when the injury occurs. Not uncommonly, the surgeon recognizes that, during his procedure, the ducts have been injured and a repair is necessary. This injury may involve either a small or a large part of the duct; it may simply consist of ligature around the duct, or it may consist of clamping or cutting part of the circumference of the duct, thus creating a defect

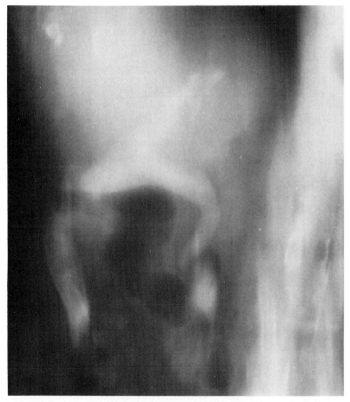

Figure 6-4 Biliary fistula. A 66 year old woman underwent a cholecystectomy for chronic cholecystitis and cholelithiasis. Two days postoperatively biliary drainage occurred around her drains. This biliary drainage persisted in amounts of 3 to 500 ml per 24 hours. An intravenous cholangiogram shows the common bile duct and the left hepatic duct. The dye is seen outlining the drain tract in the lower left corner of the photograph. The patient, diagnosed as having a possible injury to the right hepatic duct, was reoperated upon. At surgery a bile accumulation was evacuated from underneath the right lobe of the liver. The biliary fistula was found. X-rays done through the fistula revealed this to be the cystic duct. The common bile duct and hepatic ducts were found intact, and there was free flow of contrast material into the duodenum. The cause of the fistula was thought to have been a common bile duct stone that passed. This illustrates the use of intravenous cholangiography in the diagnosis of biliary fistula.

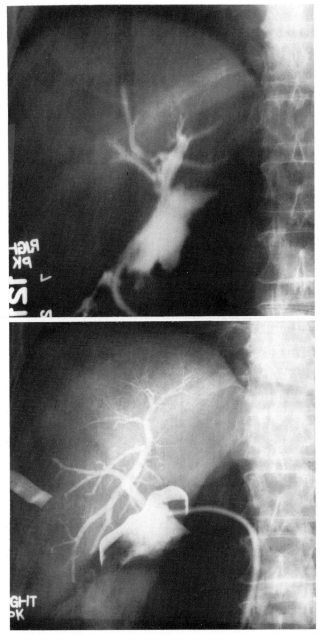

Figure 6–5   Biliary fistula. Division of both hepatic ducts. In the repair of biliary fistula resulting from bile duct injury, it is worthwhile to keep in mind that occasionally the injury involves the upper end of the hepatic duct and the ends of the individual hepatic ducts. Unless care is taken, it is possible to identify only one of the ducts and thus have a continued biliary fistula from the other lobe of the liver postoperatively. The cholangiograms illustrated here show separate right and left hepatic ducts identified during surgery for biliary fistula. The ducts were about 2 cm apart, and the injury was repaired by a hepaticojejunostomy Roux-Y, as illustrated elsewhere in this chapter. The patient is well four years later.

in the site. It may involve removal of large portions of the duct.

The simplest injury to repair at the time of primary surgery is the one involving a simple ligature of the duct in continuity and a defect in the wall of the duct not involving the entire circumference. In the case of a ligature, the ligature should be removed and a splinting T-tube inserted which bridges the area ligated. A resection of this area with reanastomosis is unnecessary, and the T-tube can be removed within a six-week period. In the case of a defect in the wall of the duct, again a T-tube needs to be inserted with closure of defect in the wall, which may necessitate mobilization of the duodenum to be able to approximate the edges of the defect in the duct wall. On rare occasions, the T-tube can be brought out through the defect, thus simplifying the repair; however, this can only be done on very small defects. Again the T-tube does not need to be left in place for more than six weeks.

The injury involving transection of the duct during operation is ideally repaired by end-to-end anastomosis at the time of injury. Unless a large segment of the duct is removed, an end-to-end anastomosis is usually feasible and is done with nonabsorbable fine suture material over a splinting T-tube, the T-tube being brought through the wall of the duct either above or below the anastomosis, depending on the length of the stump available. In this anastomosis as in other biliary enteric anastomoses, it is extremely important to avoid tension on the suture line. The duodenum should be sutured to the gallbladder fossa to avoid any tension on the suture line holding the common bile duct together. The T-tube in this instance can usually be removed in less than six months, depending on the type of injury. A bile duct injury involving the junction of the hepatic ducts or the individual hepatic ducts and discovered at surgery is probably best repaired by the use of hepaticojejunostomy, as described in the procedure for biliary fistulas.

INJURY TO BILE DUCT DURING GASTRECTOMY

A reasonably common injury to the bile duct during difficult gastrectomy involves the retroduodenal portion of the bile duct. When this injury is discovered at the time of surgery, it is important to check for a concomitant injury to the pancreatic duct. When the duodenal stump can be safely closed and there is no concomitant injury to the pancreatic duct, it is advisable to perform an end-to-side choledochoduodenostomy, with a splinting catheter emerging through the duodenum, and to remove the gallbladder at the same time. If damage to the pancreatic duct has occurred, however, con-

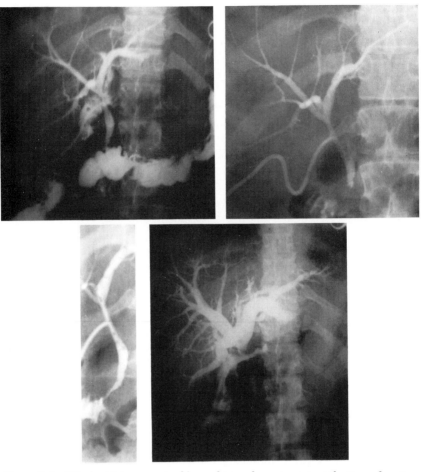

Figure 6–6   Bile duct injury repaired by end-to-end anastomosis at the time of surgery. The cholangiogram in the upper left corner is done through a T-tube immediately following end-to-end anastomosis where a small part of the bile duct has been removed with the gallbladder. The figures in the upper right corner and lower left corner are taken at intervals postoperatively prior to removal of the T-tube. The picture in lower right corner shows a stricture with dilated intrahepatic ductal system, which required repair by hepaticojejunostomy. End-to-end anastomosis for bile duct injuries done at the time of recent surgery is very likely to give good results. The anastomosis, however, should be done using nonabsorbable suture material, and where a segment of the duct has been removed, the duodenum should be suspended from the gallbladder fossa in order to avoid tension on the anastomosis. The splinting catheter should be left in place for at least six months.

sideration should be given to bringing up a Roux-Y loop of small bowel for an anastomosis to the common bile duct to avoid the occurrence of combined biliary-pancreatic fistula postoperatively. The pancreatic duct should also be reanastomosed or at least adequately drained. The gallbladder should be left in place, since it may be needed later during a predictably complicated postoperative course. Some surgeons may prefer to ligate the common duct and use the gallbladder for anastomosis associated with gastrectomy. The disadvantage of this is the probability that a biliary fistula will develop at the end of the ligated duct, since the pressure needed for filling the gallbladder through the cystic duct may be more than the ligated tissues can take. Involvement and occlusion of an intramural cystic duct by the ligature on the common bile duct can also cause development of a biliary fistula. Occlusion of the cystic duct may be avoided by demonstrating its entrance from the common duct, but the use of cholecystoenterostomy with a ligated common bile duct is likely to lead to these complications.

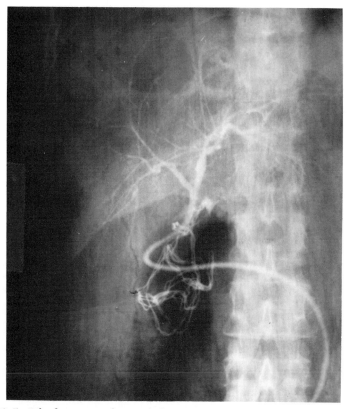

Figure 6–7   Bile duct injury during cholecystectomy. The hepatic duct and the intra-hepatic ducts are visualized through injection of contrast material via a catheter in the stump of the hepatic duct. Both hepatic ducts are easily seen, indicating that we are dealing with a single duct injury. There is a good stump of hepatic duct remaining. The distal end of the common duct could not be located, and the patient was treated with a hepaticojejunostomy Roux-Y.

THE REPAIR OF BILE DUCT INJURY BY
ROUX-Y[4] HEPATICOJEJUNOSTOMY

The choice of incision for repairs of the bile duct is often dictated by the surgeon who performed the initial surgery, since many of these patients have unhealed recent incisions. In such instances the old incision is used and enlarged. My own choice of incision is a long one extending from the left costal margin out into the right flank, parallel to the right costal margin. The hepatoduodenal ligament is approached laterally by freeing the undersurface of the right lobe of the liver from the colon and duodenum. The gallbladder fossa is usually seen first, then the descending part of the duodenum. The lymph node in the angle between the duodenum and common duct can be seen and indicates proximity to the involved area. Palpation of the hepatic artery helps to identify the hepatoduodenal ligament. When the foramen of Winslow is fused, the anterior surface of the vena cava becomes a landmark for indicating proximity to the bile duct. Once the hepatoduodenal ligament is found, the bile duct is identified by observing the leakage of bile, in the case of fistula, and by needle aspiration, in the case of stricture. Also, a nest of suture material usually is found at the level of bile duct injury, and once the sutures are found, the duct itself is near.

A cholangiogram is taken by inserting a catheter into the fistula

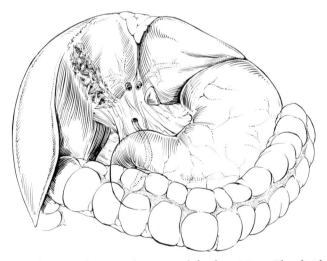

Figure 6–8 Technique of repair of common bile duct injury. The divided hepatic ducts are exposed and identified in the hilus of the liver. The ducts are further identified by injection of contrast material. (From Thorbjarnarson, B.: Repair of common bile duct injury. Surg. Gynecol. Obstet. *133*:293, 1971.)

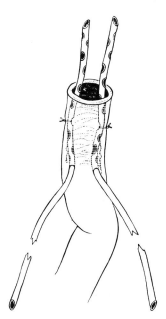

Figure 6–9 Technique of repair of common bile duct injury. Red rubber catheters are prepared as splints and for decompression of the ducts. The catheters should not fit tightly; the distance for which they are accommodated within the duct is measured. An isoperistaltic loop of jejunum is fashioned by the Roux-Y procedure, usually ante colon. The catheters, with several holes cut in the sides, are placed through separate enterostomies, and the ends are extended beyond the divided jejunum for a distance corresponding in length to the measurements already made. A chromic catgut suture is placed through the intestinal wall around the catheter at one of the side apertures. The ligature is tied down snugly, securing the catheter against displacement during the next steps in the operation or from the peristaltic action of the intestine in the postoperative period. (From Thorbjarnarson, B.: Repair of common bile duct injury. Surg. Gynecol. Obstet. *133*:293, 1971. By permission of Surgery, Gynecology and Obstetrics.)

or by injecting the contrast material through a needle. The importance of the cholangiogram is to verify the status of the ductal system above the injury and to make certain that the injury does not involve both hepatic ducts.

The hepaticojejunostomy is done in a Roux-Y fashion. The distance from the hepatic duct anastomosis to the enteroenterostomy is a little over 25 cm, and it can be either ante- or retrocolic in location. I do not believe it is necessary or advisable to dissect out a stump of the proximal bile duct. As a matter of fact, I think this is likely to interfere with the blood supply to the duct and predispose to stenosis. Likewise, I think it is unwise to place the sutures of the anastomosis into the wall of the duct for the same reasons. The open end of the bile duct fistula usually has a cuff of mucosa poking out through the tissues, and the opening represents the full diameter of the duct. In the case of strictures, the stricture and scar tissue have to be excised to create a communication to the obstructed duct, although this opening is usually of a much smaller diameter than the dilated duct itself. In the case of strictures, it is desirable to obtain an opening approaching the diameter of the dilated duct, and this can sometimes be done by longitudinal incision in the anterior wall of the duct. The anastomosis is made with silk between the surrounding tissues in the porta hepatis, with the bile duct as the central point. A splinting rubber catheter is placed through the jejunal loop about 5 cm from the end, and openings are made in the sides of the catheter. The distance to which

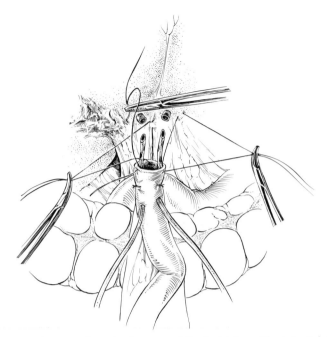

Figure 6–10   Technique of repair of common bile duct injury. The intestine is sutured around the divided ducts with silk sutures. The most important suture is the one that includes the scar tissue from the cholecystectomy. Only three sutures are placed at this time, to the right and left of the ducts and below. As these sutures are tied, the catheters are directed into the divided ends of the ducts. (From Thorbjarnarson, B.: Repair of common bile duct injury. Surg. Gynecol. Obstet. *133*:293, 1971.)

the catheter will fit inside the duct is measured and determines how far beyond the divided jejunum the catheter protrudes. The catheter is secured to the inside of the jejunum close to the end with a suture of chromic catgut that goes through the bowel wall, around the catheter, and is tied from the outside. Three sutures are placed initially between the jejunum and porta hepatis, inferiorly and on both sides. The catheter is directed into the divided duct, as the three sutures are tied down and sutures between the jejunum and porta hepatis are added as needed to complete the closure. The jejunal loop is secured to the scar tissue in the gallbladder fossa to relieve any tension, and the catheter is brought to the skin through a stab wound. Rubber drains are placed in the subhepatic space, and closure of the abdomen is undertaken.

Postoperative Care

The catheter draining the bile duct is attached to dependent drainage during the immediate postoperative period. There is usu-

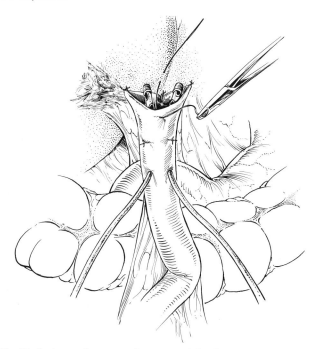

Figure 6–11 Technique of repair of common bile duct injury. With the catheters inside the ducts, the fourth, or top, suture is placed and tied down. (From Thorbjarnarson, B.: Repair of common bile duct injury. Surg. Gynecol. Obstet. *133*:293, 1971.)

ally some drainage from the rubber drains in the subhepatic space, and sometimes the drainage contains bile. The subhepatic drains are removed slowly five to seven days following surgery. Once drainage from the subhepatic space has stopped, the catheter draining the bile duct may be occluded to allow all the bile to enter the intestine and then removed within three weeks of the operation. All the patients are given antibiotics postoperatively, the specific drug being determined by the cultures of bile obtained preoperatively or during operation.

This method merits consideration first of all because of its simplicity. The anastomosis of the jejunum circumferentially in the porta hepatis is easily done and requires less time to accomplish than the traditional mucosa-to-mucosa repair. Secondly, there are few postoperative complications, probably because of the reliable drainage of the bile through the splinting catheter. The long-term results indicate that the principles advocated here, i.e., no sutures directly to the duct itself, and only a limited period of splinting of the anastomosis postoperatively, deserve consideration, particularly in the surgery of biliary fistulas. When this method is used for the

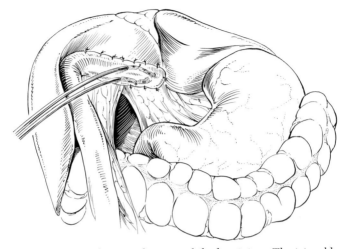

Figure 6-12   Technique of repair of common bile duct injury. The jejunal loop is now sutured to the gallbladder fossa, eliminating any tension of the four previously placed sutures. At this point, more sutures can be placed circumferentially to the end of the intestine if needed. The catheters emerge through stab wounds in the abdominal wall and are allowed to drain freely. Drains are placed down to the subhepatic space, since some bile leakage may be expected postoperatively. The decompression catheters are left in place for from three to five weeks or until bile leakage has ceased. Usually by this time the retaining catgut ligature is absorbed, and sometimes the catheter has been extruded from the common bile duct. (From Thorbjarnarson, B.: Repair of common bile duct injury. Surg. Gynecol. Obstet. *133*:293, 1971.)

relief of strictures, prolonged splinting of the anastomosis must be considered.

EVALUATION OF PATIENTS WITH BILE DUCT INJURY

Most bile duct injuries are discovered only after completion of the primary surgical procedure. The injury manifests itself either by obstructive jaundice or by prolonged, excessive bile drainage, which later may become complicated with fever, chills, and sepsis. Many of these people, particularly those who have biliary fistulas and infected subhepatic and subphrenic collections of bile, are extremely ill and need careful, prompt evaluation so that they can be brought into the optimum condition for withstanding a corrective procedure. The patient with complete mechanical obstruction is usually easy to manage, since peritonitis is not present. Cholangitis may occur in addition later, but it usually responds to the appropriate antibiotic therapy.

Patients with biliary fistulas usually have subhepatic collections of bile and on occasion may need primary drainage before any corrective procedure is begun. It is important to remember, however, that little definitive improvement can be expected in these patients unless the basic injury is corrected. Therefore, preoperative preparation should be as limited and brief as possible, mainly consisting of correction of obvious fluid and electrolyte deficiencies and of preliminary control of infection. The surgery should be undertaken at the earliest possible time and should consist of decompression of the biliary tree and biliary enteric anastomosis, in the case of strictures, and evacuation of intra-abdominal abscesses and biliary enteric anastomosis, in the case of fistulas. Because of the severe nature of the illness and the poor condition of these patients, it is of utmost importance that the surgical procedure be well planned. It should be effective enough to correct the underlying injury and yet simple enough to be carried out without exposing the patient to an unnecessarily long procedure and anesthesia.

OTHER TYPES OF DEFINITIVE OPERATIONS

Plastic Repair

On rare occasions the surgeon operating for bile duct injury may find a short, localized stricture or even a stricture involving part of the circumference of the wall of the bile duct. In these rare instances plastic closure may be undertaken. This involves a longitudinal incision with transverse closure, using fine, nonabsorbable suture material, and postoperative splinting by a T-tube emerging through an uninvolved portion of the bile duct. It must be emphasized that these situations are extremely rare.

End-to-End Anastomosis

End-to-end anastomosis is often the ideal way to correct an injury discovered at the time of the primary operation. End-to-end anastomosis can also sometimes effectively be performed for biliary fistulas when a segment of the duct has not been removed. In these cases the proximal end of the bile duct is not dilated and will fit nicely for an end-to-end anastomosis to the distal duct, again over a splinting T-tube. End-to-end anastomosis also can be done when a segment of the duct not exceeding 1 to 2 cm has been removed. In this instance mobilization of the duodenum may allow the duodenum and the pancreas to be brought up into the porta hepatis for end-to-end anastomosis of the two ductal segments. It is of extreme importance, however, to support the anastomosis by suturing the upper border of the first portion of the duodenum to the gallbladder fossa to take any tension off the anastomotic line. In the case of strictures or a ligated duct, end-to-end anastomosis becomes quite difficult and often inadvisable, since by the time surgery is undertaken, the proximal duct has undergone rather prominent dilatation and the discrepancy in size makes end-to-end anastomosis technically difficult. High strictures at the bifurcation of the hepatic duct or involving both hepatic ducts are best repaired by a Roux-Y type of hepaticojejunostomy. In the case of strictures, the scar tissue involving the ends of the ducts should be trimmed away as much as possible, and every effort should be made to have the opening into the ductal system as wide as possible. However, the anastomosis is done away from the ductal ends themselves to the surrounding liver, in contrast to the mucosa-to-mucosa anastomosis, which is done by end-to-end anastomosis of the bile duct itself.

Internal Stent

Comments have been made under the discussions of individual procedures about the use of internal stent or splints in the repair of bile duct injury. In cases in which simple transection of the duct has occurred, there is no loss of tissue, and an end-to-end anastomosis can be made at the time of the original injury, or when an end-to-end anastomosis of an injury from the transection resulting in a biliary fistula can be made, the splints usually consist of a T-tube, which needs to be left in place for only four to six weeks. When the T-tubes have been used for bridging an end-to-end anastomosis where segments of the duct have been removed and where possible tension may occur on the suture line, the stent should be left in place longer, usually up to six months or more. During this time the stent is left in to give mechanical support for the anastomosis and is only kept open in the immediate postoperative period.

The splints used in hepaticojejunostomy for biliary fistulas are best brought out through the ascending limb of the Roux-Y anastomosis in a Witzel-type fashion. They are secured at the level of anastomosis in order to provide adequate drainage in the immediate postoperative period. These splints are not left in place for long periods of time and can be removed in three to four weeks, by which time they usually have been extruded into the intestinal loop. Roux-Y anastomosis in the case of strictures is another matter. Even though success may often be obtained without long-standing use of splints, the recur-

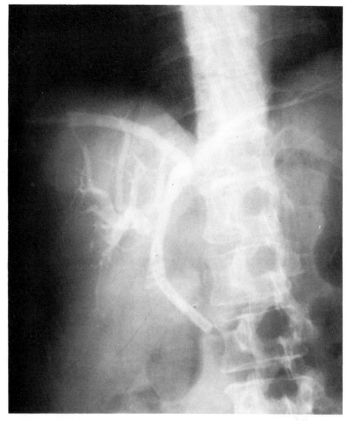

Figure 6–13 A transhepatic splint and hepaticojejunostomy. The cholangiogram is done through a transhepatic splint. The upper end comes out through the left lobe of the liver, and the lower end is free inside the ascending limb of the Roux-Y anastomosis. Transhepatic splints allow free irrigation, and if the lower end is brought out through the jejunum, the tube can be changed at will. There is often drainage around the tubes onto the skin, however, and when a straight transhepatic splint is used, as in the instance illustrated here, it is difficult to secure the tube in place and guard against accidental removal.

rence of strictures is so frequent that prolonged use of splints is advisable.

The type of splint may vary, and they may be brought to the outside in different ways. A Y-tube may be used when the bifurcation of the hepatic duct is involved, but a similar splinting may be obtained by splitting the upper end of a T-tube and putting half of the limb into each hepatic duct. The outside limb of this tube should emerge through the intestinal wall just below the anastomosis and be brought out through the abdominal wall. The use of transhepatic splints,[2] that is, straight splinting catheters that emerge through the liver parenchyma and have the lower end within the intestinal loop, has been described. These may be useful in certain circumstances, but the end coming out on the abdominal wall usually emerges in an awkward location, and there is a problem securing the end of the tube so that it does not fall out or is not pulled out by the patient inadvertently.

The reason for the use of long-standing, indwelling splints is to maintain the diameter of the anastomosis while the scar tissue matures around the anastomosis, with the hope that further contraction of the scar tissue will not occur after the tubes are removed. Thus these splints should be left in for up to 12 months before being removed. Since their main objective is to maintain the size of the anastomosis, the outside limb of the stent does not have to be hollow, although I prefer the use of the conventional T-tube splint, which enables me

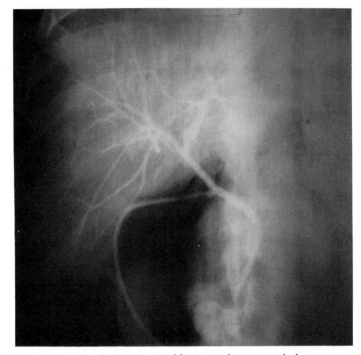

Figure 6–14 Biliary fistula. A 64 year old man underwent a cholecystectomy, which was followed by fever, jaundice, and biliary drainage to his wound. Re-exploration ten days later showed a large bile collection around the liver. The common bile duct was intact, there was no ligature on the cystic duct, and a cholangiogram done through the cystic duct shows a normal bile duct with free flow to the duodenum. The possibilities are that there was never a ligature on the cystic duct or that it slipped off. Spasm at the ampulla of Vater then directed the flow of bile into the abdominal cavity. It is also possible that a small common duct stone was present and later passed on. The patient made an uneventful recovery following his second operation. The cystic duct catheter was removed uneventfully two weeks following surgery. (See discussion of biliary fistulas, p. 150.)

to obtain dependable decompression of the ductal system in the immediate postoperative period.

IMMEDIATE RESULTS OF THE REPAIR
OF BILE DUCT INJURIES

The best results in the treatment of bile duct injuries can be expected when the proper operation is done at the earliest possible time following occurrence of injury. This means either when the injury occurs or as soon as possible thereafter. The properly performed end-to-end anastomosis at the time of injury is probably the most likely to succeed, but on the whole, considering the results of large series of bile duct injuries, the hepaticojejunostomy seems to be a safer procedure.

Morbidity and mortality are high and are directly related to the condition of the patient when he appears for the repair and the number of procedures that have been performed. At the Lahey Clinic[1] a 13 per cent mortality was reported in a large series of patients with bile duct injuries. At the same hospital they also found that 25 per cent of the patients undergoing surgery for bile duct injuries suffered complications. The main cause of postoperative morbidity is infection, but biliary fistulas and bleeding also accounted for a significant number of complications. The most common cause of death in people with bile duct injury seems to be hepatic failure, and in some of the patients this is due to acute liver failure from concomitant injury to the blood supply to the liver or from overwhelming sepsis and cholangitis. Liver failure also occurs as a late complication from gradual onset of biliary cirrhosis with portal hypertension, hemorrhage, or coma. Myocardial infarction, renal failure, and cerebral vascular accidents account for a number of fatalities following repair of bile duct injury, usually as late manifestations in patients with prolonged, severe jaundice and preceding septic complications.

LATE RESULTS OF THE REPAIR OF
BILE DUCT INJURIES

The results of surgery for bile duct injury cannot be safely predicted until at least two years have elapsed from the time of surgery. Most of the failures in surgery for bile duct injury are traced to stenosis or narrowing of the anastomosis performed either between the bile ducts themselves or between the bile duct and the intestinal tract. The occurrence of stenosis is manifested by chills, fever, and recurrent bouts of jaundice, and this is usually encountered within the first year after repair when success has not been obtained. It is quite rare to have stenosis develop in a patient who has been asymptomatic for two years following surgery, but it may occur on rare occasions. The overall success rate in the repair of bile duct injuries is about 80 per cent.[5,6] Most of these patients have only undergone one or two procedures. The success rate declines as more procedures are performed, and there are very few patients with permanent relief who have undergone more than five or six operations.[5,6] The surgery for bile duct injury is difficult, and further progress in the treatment of bile duct injuries seems to lie not in improved techniques but rather in prevention of the injury in the first place.

REFERENCES

1. Braasch, J. W.: Current considerations in the repair of bile duct strictures. Surg. Clin. North Am. 53:423, 1973.
2. Smith, R.: Hepatico-jejunostomy with transhepatic intubation for very high strictures of the hepatic duct. Br. J. Surg. 51:186, 1964.
3. Thorbjarnarson, B.: The anatomical diagnosis of jaundice by percutaneous cholangiography and its influence on treatment. Surgery 61:347, 1967.
4. Thorbjarnarson, B.: Repair of common bile duct injury. Surg. Gynecol. Obstet. 133:293, 1971.
5. Warren, K. W., Mountain, J. C., and Gray, L. W.: Use of modified Y tube splint in the repair of biliary strictures. Surg. Gynecol. Obstet. 134:665, 1972.
6. Warren, K. W., Mountain, J. C., and Midell, A. I.: Management of strictures of the biliary tract. Surg. Clin. North Am. 51:711, 1971.

Chapter Seven

TUMORS OF THE BILIARY TRACT

BENIGN TUMORS OF THE GALLBLADDER

Papillomas and adenomas are occasionally found in gallbladders removed for other reasons, particularly for stones. Elsewhere adenomyomatosis and cholesterosis of the gallbladder are discussed in some detail, and both these conditions may simulate tumor. Cholesterosis is found as a fixed filling defect on gallbladder x-rays, and adenomyomatosis is found on palpation of the fundus of the gallbladder during surgery for other causes. Papillomas and adenomas found at surgery are usually benign,[3] and a 15-year follow-up of polypoid lesions of the gallbladder diagnosed by cholecystography, failed to show any instance of gallbladder cancer developing. On the other hand, Sawyer[2] found four malignant tumors among nine grossly benign papillomas in removed gallbladders. In a review of 70 patients whose gallbladders were removed for fixed filling defects,[3] the most common histologic diagnosis was cholesterol polyp (62 per cent); the next most common were adenomyoma (24 per cent), inflammatory polyp (10 per cent), and true adenoma (4 per cent). None of the patients was found to have carcinoma.

There are few reported cases of gallbladder cancer being diagnosed by x-rays, and the question arises as to what to do when the x-ray diagnosis of a fixed filling defect is made. When symptoms compatible with gallbladder disease are present, a cholecystectomy should be advised, since a significant number of these patients, when followed over a long period of time, will be found to have stones. Patients with symptoms and cholesterosis or adenomyomatosis can

119

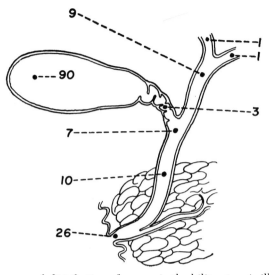

Figure 7–1 The normal distribution of cancer in the biliary tree is illustrated in this drawing describing the location of 147 biliary tree cancers. The gallbladder is by far the most common site, followed by the ampulla of Vater, the common duct, and the hepatic duct junction of hepatic and cystic ducts, in order of decreasing frequency. (From Thorbjarnarson, B., and Glenn, F.: Carcinoma of the gallbladder. Cancer *12*:1009, 1959.)

also be expected to obtain relief. At the moment, there is no convincing evidence that an asymptomatic fixed filling defect on cholecystography warrants cholecystectomy, unless change or increase in size can be demonstrated on follow-up studies.

CARCINOMA OF THE GALLBLADDER

Cancer of the biliary tree excluding the pancreas is a relatively rare disease but uncommonly deadly. It is mainly a disease of late middle and advanced age. The estimated incidence of cancer in patients operated upon for biliary disease is about 0.3 to 0.7 per cent in patients under the age of 50 and 5 to 9 per cent in patients over the age of 50. The gallbladder is the most common primary site of carcinomas of the biliary tree, and cancer is found in about one out of every 50 gallbladder operations.[19] Gallbladder cancer is more common among women than among men, in approximately the same proportion as gallstones are more common in women. Gallstones are implicated as the main cause of cancer of the gallbladder, and stones are found in at least 83 per cent of these patients. There may be an indication that stones are more important in carcinogenesis in women than in men, since 91 per cent of all women with gallbladder cancer were found also to harbor stones, whereas only 59 per cent of males were found to be similarly affected.[19] The association of stones with cancer is not fully explained. Perhaps it is long-standing chronic irritation and damage from the stones that causes the cancer,[17] but cholesterol and bile salts are closely related to compounds that have been found to cause gallbladder cancer in experimental animals.[8,9] Some indications of environmental and occupational causes of biliary tract cancer have recently been postulated.[13]

Symptoms

The symptoms and signs of gallbladder cancer vary considerably but cannot be distinguished from those of biliary tract disease caused by stones alone. The symptoms of patients with stones and cancer are usually of longer duration, averaging over five years, indicating that the stones had been present for a long time before the advent of the cancer. Patients with cancer and no stones usually have symptoms of less duration, averaging six months. The duration of symptoms does not indicate the status of the tumor. The most common symptoms in gallbladder cancer are pain, jaundice, and weight loss. Jaundice associated with gallbladder cancer is not always an unfavorable sign, although most of the time it is evidence of unresectability. A significant number of patients have concomitant common duct stones, and these rather than the tumor are causing the jaundice.

Cause of Death in Untreated Patients

Almost all patients with untreated carcinoma of the gallbladder die from liver failure secondary to outflow obstruction of the biliary tract.[10,19] As with other malignant tumors, metastatic lesions of the gallbladder can cause unusual problems; thus patients have been known to die from uremia caused by obstruction of the ureters, by metastases only discovered at autopsy, and by perforations of intra-abdominal organs due to involvement with implants and metastases. Untreated patients have not been known to live for more than a few months after the onset of severe symptoms of gallbladder tumor.[12, 19]

Diagnosis

Carcinoma of the gallbladder can only be diagnosed at surgery. Up to now there have been only isolated cases[7] of gallbladder car-

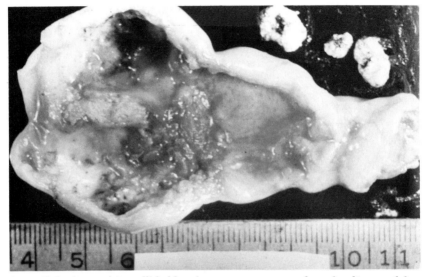

Figure 7-2 A porcelain gallbladder shows up on x-rays and can be diagnosed from plain x-rays, even though the organ is usually nonfunctioning. The gallbladder usually contains stones. There is a significantly increased incidence of cancer in porcelain gallbladders, indicating that prophylactic cholecystectomy should be carried out even in the absence of symptoms.

cinoma being diagnosed with cholecystography, but there are indications that there is a high incidence of cancer in the porcelaneous gallbladder.[4,14,15] The findings both on physical examination and through laboratory tests are the same as in calculous disease of the biliary tract, and only in the later stages, when a mass becomes palpable or distant metastases are found, do the findings vary significantly from those found in benign biliary tract disease. Most gallbladder cancers originate in the fundus of the gallbladder, but tumors originate also in the body or the ampulla of the gallbladder. These tumors and, in the later stages, those that originate in the fundus have a tendency to grow over onto the hepaticoduodenal ligament, causing obstruction of the flow of bile and jaundice. Some of the tumors in the body of the gallbladder and in the fundus, however, first cause invasion and obstruction of the duodenum or the pylorus of the stomach. Thus a reasonably early symptom may occasionally be duodenal or pyloric obstruction, even before jaundice becomes apparent.[12-19]

Pathologic Features

Most gallbladder cancers are adenocarcinomas,[6,11,19] but a small number are found to have epidermoid features. Carcinoma in situ may be diagnosed in the gallbladder, and patients with carcinoma in situ have been found to die later from metastatic lesions.[19]

Surgical Treatment

Patients undergoing surgery for gallbladder carcinoma may be divided into three groups. The first group is composed of patients with gallbladder cancers that are removed without knowledge of the presence of tumor in the gallbladder. This is not uncommon, and in this group are most of the patients who survive following removal of gallbladder cancer. If the cancer is found to be localized within the wall of the gallbladder on pathologic examination, there is probably no reason for any further surgery. The second group is made up of the patients in whom the cancer is present in the gallbladder but also invades the right lobe of the liver, where extension usually first becomes apparent. Autopsy studies in cases of gallbladder cancer have shown a small but significant number of patients dying from gallbladder cancer with the tumor still localized within the right lobe of one liver and/or growing onto the duodenal ligament and causing jaundice. This would indicate that a small number of patients might be candidates for a radical procedure involving removal of the right lobe of the liver along with the gallbladder. This procedure has been carried out on numerous occasions, but survivors are few. Still the procedure should be kept in mind in some instances.[5, 16] The third group of patients comprises those in whom distant spread and involvement of both lobes of the liver and/or involvement of the hepatic blood supply has occurred, making total removal unfeasible. Patients in this group have a very short life expectancy, but palliative procedures may make life more bearable. The symptoms that sometimes may be eased are the jaundice and associated itching. These may be helped by a T-tube placed inside the common duct, bridging the obstructed area and thus allowing bile to flow to the intestine. The duodenal and pyloric obstruction due to invasion by a cancer of the gallbladder may also be alleviated by a gastrojejunostomy.

Survival Following Surgery

Carcinoma of the gallbladder is at present the fifth most common lesion of the gastrointestinal tract and represents 3 to 4 per cent of all malignant lesions. Patients surviving for five or more years following surgery are very rare; in a series from the New York Hospital involving 90 patients, there were three seven-year survivals. All these patients had been treated by simple cholecystectomy. In this series

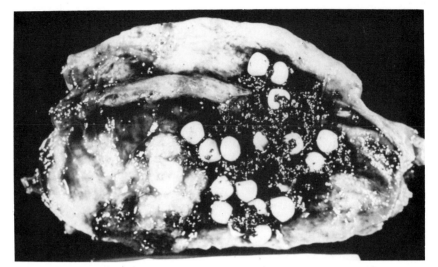

Figure 7–3 Carcinoma of the gallbladder. This acutely inflamed gallbladder containing calculi is from a patient with acute cholecystitis and common duct stones. When the gallbladder was opened in the pathology laboratory, a small tumor was found, which is seen in the lower right corner of the specimen. This tumor proved to be a carcinoma. The patient is alive and well without any sign of recurrent tumor three years since removal of this gallbladder. This is the stage at which carcinoma of the gallbladder can still be cured by simple cholecystectomy; no further operative intervention is necessary.

there were no long-term survivors following radical surgery for gall-bladder cancer. Thus at present, gallbladder cancer may be considered a universally fatal disease unless it is removed at the stage when it is not grossly recognized during surgery for benign biliary tract disorders. With 6500 persons dying from gallbladder cancer each year in the United States, it might be worthwhile to consider performing cholecystectomies in patients with asymptomatic gallstones and impressing on patients with gallstones the need for early removal. The fact that very few patients are found with gallbladder cancer before the age of 50 would set this as an obligatory age for the application of elective cholecystectomy in preventing gallbladder cancer.

CARCINOMA OF THE BILE DUCTS

Carcinoma of the bile ducts is a relatively uncommon malignant tumor, but according to Courvoisier it was observed as far back as 1508.[23] It may be found in 0.01 to 0.46 per cent of routine autopsies.[21] It is less common than carcinoma of the gallbladder, and there is probably one carcinoma of the bile duct for every three carcinomas of the gallbladder encountered on surgical services. The bile duct tumors are found in both men and women, and in some reports the majority are found in men. Whereas gallstones seem to be involved in the pathogenesis of gallbladder cancer, this does not seem to be the case in bile duct cancer, since only about one in every four patients with bile duct cancer has concomitant gallstones.[29] However, the incidence of gallstones associated with bile duct cancer has been reported to be as high as 57 per cent.[25] Bile duct cancer is found in middle aged and elderly patients and is rarely found before the age of 40. Pathologically the tumor is an adenocarcinoma, although isolated examples of sarcoma have been described.

Clinical Features

Jaundice is the single most important symptom of bile duct cancer. Progressive jaundice occurs early in the disease but may vary in intensity and fluctuate. The tumors are usually small when discovered, since the lumen of the bile duct does not allow much encroachment before it becomes obstructed. A number of other symptoms are described in association with bile duct cancer but all are insignificant compared with the occurrence of jaundice.[29] Thus some patients complain of right upper quadrant pain, and some have colicky pain. The average duration of symptoms cited in a report of 31 patients[29] with bile duct cancer was about three months. Occasionally, pruritus precedes the onset of jaundice; rarely, fever and chills indicative of cholangitis are experienced before obstruction becomes manifest by the appearance of jaundice.

Physical examination shows an enlarged liver. It is usually firm and rarely tender. When the obstructing lesion is distal to the cystic duct, the gallbladder does enlarge and become palpable, but this may also occur when the lesion is obstructing the cystic duct or the junction of the cystic duct with the hepatic duct. The gallbladder may then present as a hydrops of the gallbladder rather than as a Courvoisier's gallbladder. Laboratory examinations are important in that they show evidence of extrahepatic ductal obstruction with elevated serum bilirubin and high alkaline phosphatase. X-rays are quite unrewarding, except for percutaneous cholangiography or retrograde cannulation of the ampulla of Vater, which will be discussed in detail elsewhere.

Location

The location of bile duct carcinomas seems to be directly related to the length and size of the individual components of the biliary

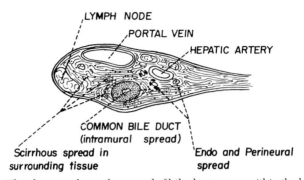

Figure 7–4   This drawing shows the spread of bile duct cancer within the bile duct and the hepaticoduodenal ligament. The reason for poor results in resection of bile duct cancer is obvious. (From Thorbjarnarson, B.: Carcinoma of the bile ducts. Cancer *12*:708, 1959.)

ductal system. Thus they are most commonly found in the common duct, that is, from the cystic duct down to the ampulla of Vater. Less frequently they are found in the hepatic duct, in the junction of the cystic duct and the bile ducts, and in the cystic duct itself or the individual hepatic ducts.

Pathologic Findings

These tumors are usually small when they are found, because jaundice develops early in the course of the disease, bringing the patient to the attention of the surgeon. At operation, the tumors are usually found infiltrating the ductal system. When located in the parts of the ductal system outside the liver parenchyma, they are found either as intraluminal papillomatous growths (which, however, is a rare occurrence) or, more commonly, as infiltrating scirrhous neoplasms spreading widely up and down the walls of the bile ducts from the primary growth, which often may be found by external palpation. There is usually irregular involvement of the duct, creating a nodular appearance, which at times has been appropriately described as palpating a string of beads. Distant metastases are found in only half the patients with primary bile duct carcinoma at the time of surgery, and even at autopsy there is a significant number of patients who still exhibit a localized tumor.[29] When metastases occur, the most common sites are the liver and regional lymph nodes, followed by the peritoneum and distant lymph nodes. Invasion of the hepatico-duodenal ligament may occur fairly early, and tumor spread is found in the endo- and perineural spaces in the ligament. In addition there is direct invasion of the areolar tissues surrounding the portal vein.

Direct invasion of the hepatic artery and portal vein is common and constitutes the most common evidence of incurability.

The tumors involving the intrahepatic portions of the bile ducts are more difficult to demonstrate at the time of operation. However, once they have reached some size, there is usually hardness over the dome of the liver where the tumor is residing, and on exploration of the ducts, resistance and obstruction may be demonstrated by both probing and x-ray. Some of these tumors are papillomatous, as mentioned earlier. These sometimes originate inside the hepatic radices, and on occasion a piece of tumor tissue may become detached and fall into the common bile duct, causing obstruction distally.[30] When this occurs it is important to retrieve the piece of tumor and have it subjected to histologic examination, since this may establish the diagnosis. The histologic diagnosis at the time of surgery may be difficult to establish, particularly when the tumors are residing high up in the ductal system at or above the bifurcation, since direct biopsy through the wall is difficult in these areas. The diagnosis can usually be established, however, by a full-thickness biopsy of the wall of the thickened and hardened duct. If the wall does not seem to be involved, then curetting of the area of obstruction with a sharp instrument through the lumen of the bile duct may yield proof of the diagnosis.

The malignant tumors of the biliary tree or ductal system are mainly adenomacarcinomas.[21] Other types of tumor may be found, such as the papillomatous type, and there is a possibility that some of these cancers originate in preexisting benign papillomas of the ductal system. That this is a common etiologic factor is not likely, since the benign papillomas of the biliary tree are rare. There are cases on record, however, in which papillomatosis of the ductal system has been found to lead to carcinoma of the bile duct, and papillomas of the bile duct with carcinomatous changes have been described.[22] Only rarely are epidermoid carcinomas and other rare types of tumors, such as adenoacanthomas, found.

Surgical Treatment

Most patients with bile duct cancer are incurable, and have tumors that are unresectable, when they are seen by the surgeon. The reasons for unresectability or incurability are usually invasion of the hepatic artery and portal vein or involvement of the tumor at the bifurcation of the hepatic ducts, with the tumor in both lobes of the liver. A significant number of patients also have distant metastases at the time of operation.[29] The resectability of the lesions is usually under 20 per cent, and most of the resectable ones involve the distal

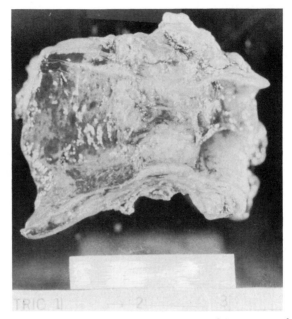

Figure 7–5 Carcinoma of the common bile duct treated by segmental resection and hepaticojejunostomy. The bile duct is open and the tumor is in its middle, somewhat more towards the right end of the specimen. Carcinomas of the bile duct usually spread extensively intramurally in the bile ducts. As might be expected this patient developed obstructive jaundice from a recurrence six months after her primary operation.

part of the bile duct, where they are removed by pancreaticoduodenectomy using the Whipple procedure.[21,29] The surgery and procedures employed may be divided into curative procedures and palliative procedures. The curative procedure to be considered is right or left hepatic lobectomy, which is suitable for certain types of hepatic duct cancer, proximally in the right and left hepatic ducts. The tumors involving the junction of the cystic and hepatic ducts may be removed by local resection and by either end-to-end anastomosis of the bile duct or hepaticojejunostomy.[24] Distal to the cystic duct, the tumors are removed by pancreaticoduodenotomy; most of the long-term survivors are found in this group.

Palliative Procedures

Palliation from symptoms of bile duct cancer usually revolves around relief of the jaundice and its concomitant pruritus, which at times may be quite severe. The procedures available for decompression of the intrahepatic bile ducts are drainage of the ducts through

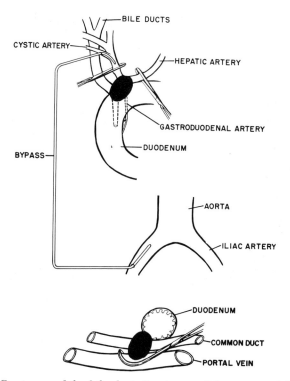

Figure 7–6 Carcinoma of the bile duct. Carcinoma of the common bile duct at the upper border of the duodenum is particularly apt to involve the portal vein and the hepatic artery, even early in its course. The drawing illustrates a method used for removal of such tumors. It involves an arterial shunt from the iliac artery through the cystic artery into the hepatic artery, resection of the hepatic artery with end-to-end anastomosis, and tangential resection of the portal vein with repair of the defect without complete division of the vein.

splinting tubes crossing the tumorous area, anastomosis of jejunum to the right or left hepatic ducts above the level of obstruction, and resection of part of the lobe of the liver with anastomosis of the bile ducts in the resected area to a loop of jejunum.[26,28] Simple drainage to the outside through a catheter placed through the substance of the liver into the bile duct can also be performed, particularly if pruritus is the main symptom and biliary intestinal anastomosis is not feasible. Decompression of the liver through a splinting T-tube has given good results in a significant number of patients. Since some of these tumors are relatively slow-growing, numerous cases are on record in which patients have lived for years with simple decompression of this type.[29,30] Jaundice can be alleviated and pruritus overcome by drainage of only one lobe of the liver for palliation, and when the obstruction involves the bifurcation of the ducts, usually only one

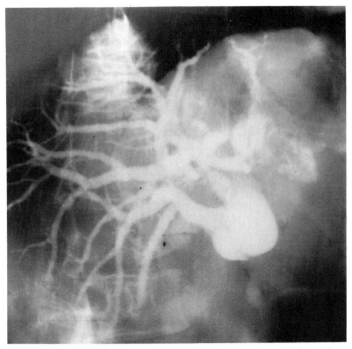

Figure 7-7   Carcinoma of the hepatic duct. The percutaneous cholangiogram shows a complete obstruction in the mid common hepatic duct. The rounded edges indicate that this is a carcinoma.

lobe should be drained.[30] The proximal end of the tube is placed into the dilated part of the hepatic duct after first dilating the carcinomatous stricture to allow passage of the tube. If the lower part of the bile duct is uninvolved with tumor, the tube can reside entirely within the ductal system. When there is extensive infiltration of the extrahepatic ductal system, it may be advisable to have a long arm extending through the ampulla of Vater into the duodenum for drainage purposes. The insertion of these tubes is usually fairly simple, since only rarely is there complete occlusion of the bile duct from the carcinomatous growth. Usually it is only occluded by pressure from the scirrhous growth within the walls of the duct but not necessarily breaking through the mucosa. A fine probe can usually be passed up the duct, then the duct sequentially dilated with enlarging size bougies until the T-tube can be placed. A hepaticojejunostomy, that is, Roux-Y anastomosis of the jejunum to the right and left hepatic ducts, when it can be done, is preferred to splinting by a T-tube, since there is no outside drainage and the patient is saved the discomfort of external dressings and of drainage from a tube emerging onto the skin.

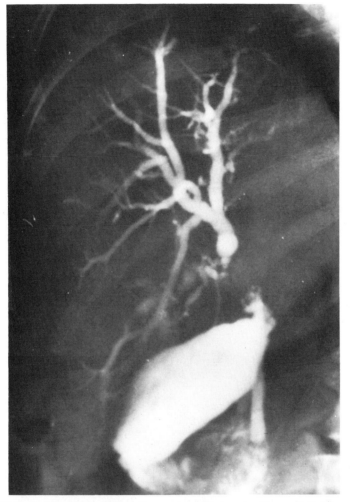

Figure 7–8 A delayed film from the same patient as in Figure 7–7. The contrast material has now passed through the obstruction. It has filled the distal bile duct and the gallbladder. The area involved by tumor is easily seen; it ranges from the level of the cystic duct to the upper part of the common hepatic duct. Jaundice may at times be intermittent in carcinoma of the bile ducts and ampulla of Vater. The complete obstruction is then probably caused by cellular debris or mucous plugs, which at times may be flushed out with complete or partial disappearance of the jaundice. This patient was treated by cholecystectomy and T-tube drainage across the tumor. She survived for one year following the operation, then died from liver failure.

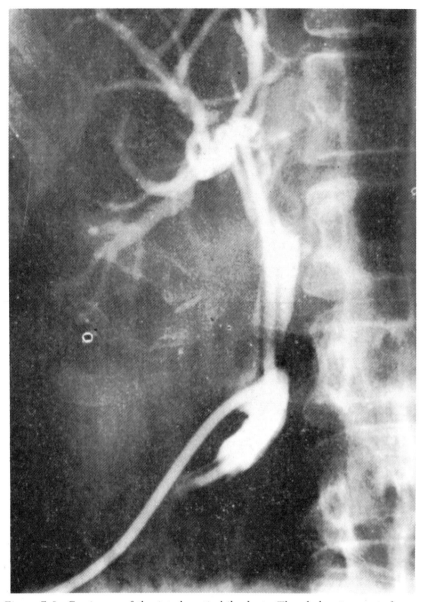

Figure 7–9 Carcinoma of the intrahepatic bile ducts. The cholangiogram is from a
54 year old woman with carcinoma of the left main hepatic duct invading and compress-
ing the right hepatic duct and thus causing jaundice. The cholangiogram shows an
indwelling T-tube bridging the obstructed area and entering the right hepatic duct.
This patient lived for seven years with an indwelling T-tube but ultimately died from
widespread metastases. (From Thorbjarnarson, B.: Carcinoma of the intrahepatic
ducts. Arch. Surg. 77:908, 1958. Copyright 1958, The American Medical Association.)

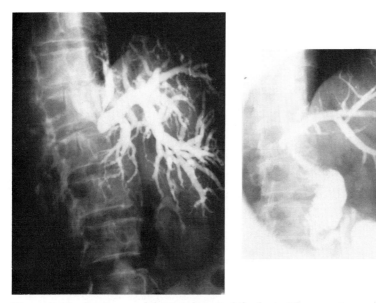

Figure 7–10 Carcinoma of the intrahepatic bile ducts. The percutaneous cholangiogram on the left shows a greatly dilated left hepatic ductal system. There is a trickle of contrast material into the right hepatic duct. At surgery a large carcinoma originating in the right hepatic duct and involving the left hepatic duct was found unresectable. The right half of the picture shows a Roux-Y loop of jejunum that has been brought up to the left hepatic duct for anastomosis. The indwelling splinting catheter is also seen on the x-ray. The patient lived for one year following the operation and died from liver failure.

Results of Surgery

The results of surgery for bile duct cancer are poor. Isolated reports cite a few patients alive after radical procedures.[20, 21] There is a fairly high mortality from the procedures themselves, particularly from the radical resections such as hepatic lobectomy or pancreaticoduodenectomy. A report by Braasch from the Lahey Clinic cites a 25 per cent mortality in pancreaticoduodenectomy for lesions of the lower end of the common duct;[21] other series report a lower mortality.[20] In a series from the New York Hospital, only 14 per cent of patients were found to have resectable lesions at the time of surgery. There was only one long-term survivor following resection of tumor, but several patients survived up to two years following insertion of a T-tube without removal of the lesion.[29] Chemotherapy and x-ray therapy have been tried with unresectable tumors of the bile ducts. Information is scanty, and no clear-cut results have been seen in patients on this therapy. Possibly individual patients may benefit from local radiation or chemotherapy, administered either through hepatic artery infusion or systemically.[21]

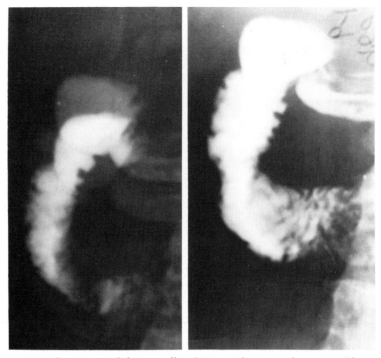

Figure 7–11 Carcinoma of the ampulla of Vater. The x-ray shows spot films of the duodenum of a patient with obstructive jaundice. There is a filling defect and an impression on the junction of the second and third portions of the duodenum.

CARCINOMA OF THE AMPULLA OF VATER

Malignant neoplasms involving the ampulla of Vater, excluding those that arise in the pancreas, have a relatively favorable prognosis as compared to other cancers of the pancreatic-biliary tree area. The periampullary tumors are rare neoplasms. They occur about as frequently as do carcinomas of the bile ducts, but carcinoma of the gallbladder and carcinoma of the pancreas are still by far the most common neoplasms of the pancreatic-biliary tree area. Carcinoma of the ampulla of Vater is more common among males than among females and in this way is similar to carcinoma of the bile ducts.[36,40]

Diagnosis

The diagnosis of carconoma of the ampulla of Vater is difficult in the early stages, since the clinical course is usually characterized by

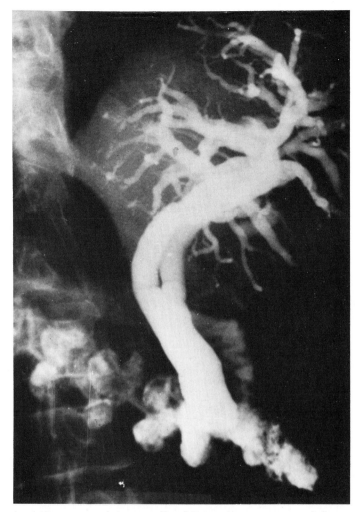

Figure 7–12 Carcinoma of the ampulla of Vater. A percutaneous cholangiogram of the same patient as in Figure 7–11 shows a greatly dilated biliary ductal system with a smooth, rounded obstruction at the lower end of the duct. The lower end of the duct is partly obscured by barium in the colon.

an insidious weight loss and mild gastrointestinal symptoms. Usually only the onset of jaundice, which is sometimes intermittent,[37] is an indication of the real problem. The onset of jaundice is often late in the course of ampullary carcinomas, since commonly the tumor breaks down and thus prevents complete biliary obstruction for a significant period of time; sometimes cholangitis accompanies the jaundice.[38] Commonly there is mild bleeding from the tumor in the ampulla, and the presence of occult blood in the stools serves to alert

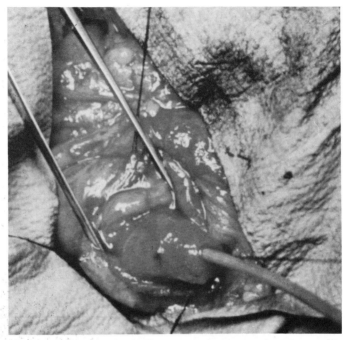

Figure 7–13 Carcinoma of the ampulla of Vater. A photograph of the ampulla of Vater in the same patient as in Figure 7–11. The duodenum has been opened up, and the ampulla of Vater is brought into view with a bougie emerging through the sphincter of Oddi. The ampulla is large and prominent, explaining the filling defect on the x-rays. There is no tumor on the duodenal side of the ampulla.

the physician to the possible presence of an ampullary carcinoma. Weight loss has usually been evident for a considerable time prior to the onset of jaundice. This weight loss is caused by impaired nutrition secondary to partial biliary and pancreatic obstruction. Rarely, steatorrhea is evident, but mild malabsorption is not uncommon, and sometimes mild forms of diabetes, probably related to pancreatitis secondary to pancreatic ductal obstruction, are discovered at the time of hospitalization. Findings on physical examination are usually unrewarding except for the presence of jaundice and the demonstration of a distended gallbladder and an enlarged liver.

Laboratory findings that help in diagnosing carcinoma of the ampulla are the presence of occult blood in the stools, evidence of obstructive jaundice, a mild degree of pancreatic insufficiency with perhaps recent onset of diabetes, and occasionally the demonstration of steatorrhea. Radiologic examination is rarely diagnostic for an ampullary tumor. In a recent series from the Lahey Clinic, 30 per cent of patients with ampullary carcinomas were found to have positive findings on upper gastrointestinal series;[39] this was also found to be true in a similar number of patients from the New York Hospital.[36] Rarely, patients with ampullary carcinoma are diagnosed prior to the onset of jaundice. Usually these patients complain of abdominal pain, upper gastrointestinal disturbances, and occasionally fever and chills, and further investigation reveals pancreatitis, elevated serum amylase, and almost always elevation of alkaline phosphatase as evidence of early bile duct obstruction. Further investigation of ampullary tumors may now be done by duodenoscopy, which allows direct inspection of the ampulla, and by retrograde cannulation with cholangiogram, if need be. Cytologic examination of duodenal aspirate is rarely helpful in establishing a diagnosis of malignant tumor of the ampulla. More often, direct biopsy of the ampulla through the duodenoscope establishes the diagnosis.

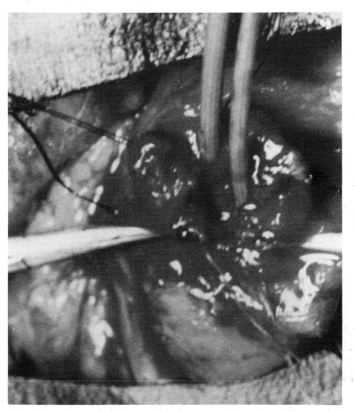

Figure 7–14 Carcinoma of the ampulla of Vater. When the sphincter of Oddi was opened, a small tumor was found in the very distal part of the ampulla of Vater. An amputation of the ampulla of Vater with reimplantation of the common bile duct and the pancreatic duct was done. This photograph shows part of the procedure, with catheters in the common bile duct and in the pancreatic duct. The patient recovered but died a year and a half later from carcinoma of the colon.

Pathology

The lesion involving the ampulla of Vater can arise from either the bile duct or the duodenal epithelium, and it may be possible to demonstrate this on microscopic examination.[36] Grossly the tumors present as polypoid growths, replacing the papilla of Vater, or as an ulcer involving the same area. Rarely there is only enlargement and firmness of the papilla, with the tumor invading from within the ampulla. Still more rarely, the lesion extends around the duodenum or directly invades the pancreas.[36] Invasion of the pancreas is directly related to the size of the tumor, which is usually small. In the series from the New York Hospital, half the tumors were 3 cm or less in diameter, and only three of these small tumors invaded the pancreas. Metastases occur late in ampullary cancer; they are usually limited to the peripancreatic nodes but may on occasion be disseminated.

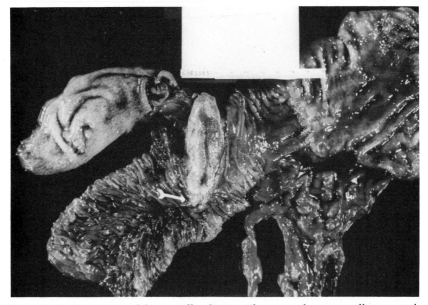

Figure 7–15 Carcinoma of the ampulla of Vater. The arrow shows a small tumor at the duodenal end of the ampulla of Vater. The bile duct and attached gallbladder, duodenum, and stomach to the right demonstrate the extent of resection for carcinoma of the ampulla of Vater. The head of the pancreas is behind the duodenum and the bile duct. This patient's symptoms were primarily those of recurrent pancreatitis and cholangitis. She is alive and well six years following radical pancreaticoduodenectomy.

Radical Pancreaticoduodenectomy for Carcinoma of the Ampulla and Lower End of the Common Duct

The Whipple operation was first described as a two-stage operation in 1935.[40] At present, it is usually done in one stage with some modifications. The abdominal incisions used for the Whipple procedure may vary. Bilateral subcostal incision gives excellent exposure and is probably the incision of choice in patients with a wide costal angle who are on the heavy side. A right paramedial incision or a midline incision is quite adequate in thin patients. The incisions must be generous since proper exposure is of paramount importance. Exploration of the abdomen and determination of resectability include examination of the liver and paraduodenal and lesser sack lymph nodes. The demonstration of metastases in the liver or lesser sack lymph nodes indicates incurability, and radical operation is then inadvisable. When the lymph nodes and liver are not involved, the next step is to investigate the relationship of the tumor to the portal vein and the hepatic artery.

A preliminary idea of involvement of the portal vein is obtained by incising the peritoneal reflexion of the duodenum and rotating the duodenum and the head of the pancreas medially (Kocher maneuver). The portal vein can now be exposed under the common bile duct, demonstrating whether or not it is involved above the pancreas. Next the lesser omental sack should be opened through the gastrohepatic omentum and the hepatic artery exposed. The gastroduodenal artery is ligated and divided. This allows exposure of the hepatic artery to the point where it curves up into the hepatoduodenal ligament, and any tumor involvement can be ascertained. Finally, the duodenum is followed and the superior mesenteric vein exposed as it crosses the duodenum on its way into the groove between the uncinate process and the body of the pancreas. To obtain adequate exposure of this part of the vein, either the omentum is removed from the transverse colon or the gastrocolic omentum is divided and the lesser sack opened. The right gastroepiploic vein runs from the greater curvature to the superior mesenteric vein at its junction with the splenic vein. The gastroepiploic vein should be secured at this point before the portal vein is exposed, since it is thin-walled and may easily be torn, causing troublesome bleeding. The superior mesenteric vein can now be exposed on its anterior surface up to the inferior border of the pancreas, and the fingers may be passed between the pancreas and the vein from above and below to demonstrate freedom from invasion. The stomach is then divided at its middle and the part to be removed rotated over to the patient's right side. The body of the pancreas is now exposed and can be divided just to the left of the tunnel created by the portal vein. There are marginal

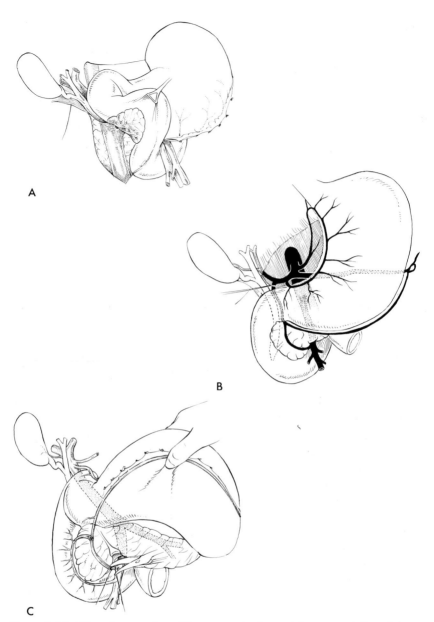

A

B

C

Figure 7–16 Whipple procedure. Three steps in determining resectability of tumors of the ampulla and lower common bile duct. (A) By doing the Kocher maneuver the surgeon can visualize the lower part of the common bile duct and portal vein. Encroachment on the portal vein by bile duct tumor can be detected here. Moreover, an approximate idea of the relationship of the tumor to the mesenteric vessels can be obtained by palpation. (B) When the lesser omental sack is entered through the gastrohepatic omentum, the gastroduodenal artery may be identified and secured. The earliest invasion of the hepatic artery from these tumors occurs here. (C) After reflecting and dividing the transverse mesocolon off the second and third portions of the duodenum, the superior mesenteric vein is exposed. The vein is followed as it disappears under the pancreas. It is most important to identify and divide the right gastroepiploic vein as illustrated, since it is easily torn and can cause troublesome bleeding.

140

vessels in the pancreas, and these may be secured by suture ligatures before division. When the pancreas is divided, a note is made of the location of the pancreatic duct. The duct is usually toward the anterior surface of the body of the pancreas. The stomach and pancreas are now brought to the patient's right side, exposing the portal vein and the junction with the splenic vein. The common bile duct is freed from the hepatic artery. The ligament of Treitz is divided and the duodenum freed from beneath mesenteric vessels. This is best done by approach above and below the transverse mesocolon and underneath the small bowel mesentery. The duodenum is divided at the ligament of Treitz. Many small veins going from the head of the pancreas and uncinate process to the superior mesenteric vein are secured, and the pancreas is then separated from the retroperitoneal tissues between clamps placed parallel to the portal vein. At the upper border of the pancreas, the pyloric vein sometimes is separately identified and secured. The specimen now is attached only by the bile duct. Next the gallbladder is removed from the liver, and once the cystic duct is free, the hepatic duct is divided. The gallbladder and common bile duct are removed with the tumor.

Reconstruction is performed by bringing the first part of the jejunum through the rent in the transverse mesocolon. The end of the jejunum is anastomosed end-to-end to the pancreas with two layers of silk sutures telescoping the divided end of the pancreas into the jejunum. I prefer to leave a splinting tube (No. 16 polyethylene tube) in the pancreatic duct and bring it through the jejunum and abdominal wall for drainage. The hepatic duct is anastomosed end-to-side to the jejunum about 6 inches from the pancreatic anastomosis. The duct is decompressed either by a small T-tube emerging from the duct or by a small red rubber tube emerging from the jejunum. Reconstruction is completed by an antecolic isoperistaltic Polya gastrojejunostomy. A vagectomy is done when there is a suspicion of concomitant ulcer disease.

Invasion of the portal vein or hepatic artery by tumor is probably a contraindication to surgical removal. However, on occasion a tangential section of the portal vein can be removed without sacrificing it altogether; similarly, a small segment of the hepatic artery can be removed and the artery reconstituted by an end-to-end anastomosis or a graft. Reports are still uncertain and remain to be proved.

There is controversy about the handling of the pancreatic stump in the Whipple procedure. It has been indicated by some authors that the pancreatic duct can be ligated and the gland allowed to atrophy. It has been our experience, however, that, when the pancreatic parenchyma is largely intact and the duct not completely obstructed by tumor, such as may happen in tumors of the lower end of the common duct and in ampullary lesions, there is risk of pancreatic cyst or fistula formation when drainage is not provided.

Postoperative Complications

Complications following the Whipple procedure are fairly common. Significant complications are encountered in from 25 to 33 per cent of operations performed.[32, 39] The most common complication directly related to the type of surgery is pancreatic fistula, which may occur in up to 12 per cent of operations.[39] Postoperative hemorrhage is not uncommon and is usually from the area of the pancreaticojejunostomy, but it has also occurred from the choledochojejunostomy and the retroperitoneum. Hemorrhage is commonly seen with a pancreatic fistula and is probably related to digestion by the pancreatic ferments. Biliary fistulas occur occasionally in the bile duct anastomosis, but both the pancreatic and biliary fistulas usually close spontaneously as long as adequate drainage has been provided. A late complication of the Whipple procedure is the development of a jejunal ulcer, which is reported to have developed in 7.5 per cent of patients in a large series from the Lahey Clinic.[39] Some surgeons prefer to do a vagectomy as an adjunct to the operation to avoid marginal ulcer, and certainly this should be done when there is pre-existing ulcer disease. Pancreatic insufficiency is fairly common but usually not severe. Mild diabetes and malabsorption usually respond well to insulin and pancreatic enzyme supplement. Although it is difficult to demonstrate patency of pancreaticojejunostomy at post-mortem examination several years following surgery, it is my impression that less pancreatic supplements are needed and that malabsorption is less of a problem when the pancreas has been anastomosed to the intestine than when the duct has been ligated and the pancreas left detached. Patients seen with pseudocyst following closure of the pancreatic stump during Whipple operations have improved their absorption dramatically following anastomosis of the cyst to the intestine.

Mortality

Mortality from the Whipple operation has been high but shows signs of falling.[34] A cumulative review up to 1965[34] showed an overall mortality of 21.3 per cent. This mortality fell to 16.2 per cent, according to a cumulative review for the five years 1965 to 1969.[32] Selected reports of large numbers of Whipple resections without mortality have also been published.[39] Carcinoma of the ampulla of Vater is usually the easiest lesion to remove by pancreaticoduodenectomy and should thus have the lowest operative mortality. This seems to be supported by the two reviews quoted above, in which 140 resections done between 1965 and 1969 had a mortality of only 9.3 per cent.[32]

Long-term Survival

Carcinoma of the ampulla of Vater has the best prognosis of all biliary tract cancers. Long-term survival is fairly common, and five-year survival is seen in over 35 per cent of patients undergoing resection.[31,32,36,38]

The long-term survivors of the Whipple operation may suffer some side effects from their operation. Commonly, pancreatic ferment must be given orally to improve fat digestion. The need for pancreatic supplements seems to be much less among patients who have their pancreases reanastomosed to the intestinal tract, and a large number of these patients do not need supplements at all. Diabetes is not uncommon among long-term survivors, but usually it was evident in some form before the operation; the severity of the diabetes may be in some way related to the degree of pancreatitis preoperatively and found at operation. Several late postoperative deaths have been related to marginal ulcer with bleeding or perforation. This complication has focused attention on the need for an adequate gastrectomy as part of the procedure and for the addition of vagectomy when ulcer was present at operation or there was a history of ulcer disease.

REFERENCES

1. Eelkema, H. H., Hodpson, J. R., and Stauffer, M. H.: Fifteen year follow-up of polypoid lesions of the gallbladder diagnosed by cholecystography. Gastroenterology 42:144, 1962.
2. Sawyer, K. C.: The unrecognised significance of papillomas, polyps and adenomas of the gallbladder. Am. J. Surg. 120:570, 1970.
3. Selzer, D. W., Dockerty, M. B., Stauffer, M. H., and Priestly, J. T.: Papillomas in the noncalculous gallbladder. Am. J. Surg. 103:472, 1962.
4. Beck, R. N., et al.: Carcinoma in the porcellain gallbladder. Radiology 106:29, 1973.
5. Brasfield, R. D.: Right hepatic-lobectomy for carcinoma of gallbladder. Ann. Surg. 153:563, 1961.
6. Carpenter, Y., et al.: Primary sarcoma of the gallbladder. Cancer 32:493, 1973.
7. Clemett, A. R., and Gould, H. R.: Polypoid gallbladder carcinoma on I.V. cholangiogram. Comtemp. Surg. 4:61, 1974.
8. Fortner, J.: Experimental induction of primary carcinoma of the gallbladder. Cancer 8:687, 1955.
9. Fortner, J., and Randall, H.: On the carcinogenity of human gallstones. Surg. Forum 12:155, 1961.
10. Havstrom, L., et al.: The natural history of primary and secondary malignant tumors of the liver. Arch. Clin. Scand. 139:264, 1973.
11. Higgs, W. R., et al.: Malignant mixed tumors of the gallbladder. Cancer 32:471, 1973.
12. Keill, R. H., and De Weese, M. S.: Primary carcinoma of the gallbladder. Am. J. Surg. 125:726, 1973.
13. Krain, L. S.: Gallbladder and extrahepatic bile duct carcinoma. Geriatrics 27:111, 1972.
14. Polk, H. C., Jr.: Carcinoma and the calcified gallbladder. Gastroenterology 50:582, 1966.

15. Rogers, L. F.: Calcifying mucinous adenocarcinoma of the gallbladder. Am. J. Gastroenterol. 59:441, 1973.
16. Pack, G. T., Miller, T. R., and Brasfield, R. D.: Total right hepatic-lobectomy for carcinoma of gallbladder. Ann. Surg. 142:6, 1955.
17. Petrov, N. N., and Krotkina, N. A.: Experimental carcinoma of the gallbladder. Ann. Surg. 125:241, 1947.
18. Tanja, M. R., and Ewing, J. B.: Primary malignant tumors of the gallbladder. Surgery 67:418, 1970.
19. Thorbjarnarson, B., and Glenn, F.: Carcinoma of the gallbladder. Cancer 12:1009, 1959.
20. Aston, S. J., and Longmire, W. P., Jr.: Pancreaticoduodenal resection: Twenty years' experience. Arch. Surg. 106:813, 1973.
21. Braasch, J. W., Warren, K. W., and Kune, G. A.: Malignant neoplasms of the bile ducts. Surg Clin. North Am. 47:627, 1967.
22. Cattell, R. B., Braasch, J. W., and Kahn, F.: polypoid epithelial tumors of the bile duct. New Engl. J. Med. 266:57, 1962.
23. Courvoisier, L. C.: Casuistisch-Statistische Beitrage zur Pathologie und chirurgie der Gallenwege. Leipzig, F. C. W. Vogel, 1890.
24. Klippel, A. P., Shaw, R. B.: Carcinoma of the common bile duct. Arch. Surg. 104:102, 1972.
25. Neibling, H. A., Dockerty, M. B., and Waugh, J. M.: Carcinoma of the extrahepatic bile ducts. Surg. Gynecol. Obstet. 89:429, 1949.
26. Ragins, H., Diamond, A., and Meny, C. H.: Intrahepatic cholangio-jejunostomy in the management of malignant biliary obstruction. Surg. Gynecol. Obstet. 136:27, 1973.
27. Sako, K., Seitzinger, G. I., and Garside, E.: Carcinoma of the extrahepatic bile duct. Surgery 41:416, 1957.
28. Sargent, R. F., Wilson, S. D., and Kaufman, H. M.: Bilateral cholangio-jejunostomy for sclerosing carcinoma of the intrahepatic bile ducts. Am. J. Surg. 123:729, 1972.
29. Thorbjarnarson, B.: Carcinoma of the bile ducts. Cancer 12:708, 1959.
30. Thorbjarnarson, B.: Carcinoma of the intrahepatic bile ducts. Arch. Surg. 77:908, 1958.
31. Aston, S. J., and Longmire, W. P., Jr.: Pancreaticoduodenal resection. Twenty years' experience. Arch. Surg. 106:813, 1973.
32. Beall, W. S., Dyer, H. A., and Stephenson, H. E.: Disappointments in the management of patients with malignancies of pancreas, duodenum and common bile duct. Arch. Surg. 101:461, 1970.
33. Blumgard, L. H., and Kennedy, A.: Carcinoma of the ampulla of Vater and duodenum. Br. J. Surg. 60:33, 1973.
34. Child, C. G., and Frey, C. F.: Pancreatico-duodenectomy. Surg. Clin. North Am. 46:1201, 1966.
35. Howard, J. M.: Pancreatico-duodenectomy: Forty-one consecutive Whipple resections without an operative mortality. Ann. Surg. 168:629, 1968.
36. Moody, F., and Thorbjarnarson, B.: Carcinoma of the ampulla of Vater. Am. J. Surg. 107:572, 1964.
37. Oliai, A., et al.: Disappearance and prolonged absence of jaundice and hyperbilirubinemia in carcinoma of the ampulla of Vater. Am. J. Gastroenterol. 59:518, 1973.
38. Ponka, J. L., and Uthappa, N. S.: Carcinoma of the ampulla of Vater. Am. J. Surg. 121:263, 1971.
39. Warren, K. W., Veidenheimer, M. C., and Pratt, H. S.: Pancreato-duodenectomy for periampullary cancer. Surg. Clin. North Am. 47:639, 1967.
40. Whipple, A. O., Parsons, W. B., and Mullins, C. R.: Treatment of carcinoma of ampulla of Vater. Ann. Surg. 102:763, 1935.

Chapter Eight

COMPLICATIONS OF
BILIARY TRACT
SURGERY

The history of planned biliary tract surgery probably starts with J. Marion Sims' cholecystostomy in April, 1878.[6] His patient died eight days later from massive hemorrhage, undoubtedly brought on by lack of vitamin K assimilation, since long-standing obstructive jaundice had been present. Thus the first planned operation on the biliary tract ended in failure because of a postoperative complication. As experience has been gained, a number of complications have become recognized as particular to biliary tract surgery. Some of these, such as bleeding from lack of vitamin K assimilation, have been almost entirely overcome; others are still with us.

The complications of biliary tract surgery may be divided into two main groups. The larger group includes complications that might be anticipated before the operation. These may be associated with the preoperative preparation of the patient, the technique and performance of the operation itself, or coexisting infirmities related or unrelated to the biliary tract disease. The smaller group includes complications that could not have been anticipated but still occur frequently enough to warrant close observation. Many of the complications that can be anticipated can also be avoided. This involves the areas of accurate diagnosis, careful preoperative and postoperative preparation of the patient, and meticulous surgery.[7]

Surgeons have observed a decrease in both morbidity and mortality over the past 40 years. This is due to improvement in diagnosis, better facilities for both preoperative and postoperative care, and the proper training of young surgeons in biliary tract surgery. The results

145

of biliary tract surgery have never been better than at present. This should not make us satisfied with the status quo, however, since the incidence of complications that can be anticipated is still considerable and there is room for improvement.

SUBHEPATIC ACCUMULATIONS AND ABSCESSES

Following the completion of biliary tract surgery, the liver, especially its right lobe, overlies the operative area. In the space between the right lobe of the liver and the transverse mesocolon there is normally some accumulation of blood, bile, and tissue fluids, but only occasionally does this accumulation become severe enough to cause trouble. Drains are normally placed in the subhepatic area following surgery. These drains should be twisted on the second postoperative day and then gradually removed, unless an abscess has been drained, in which case the drains are left in longer. Every once in a while, however, the drains fail to serve their purpose, and an accumulation becomes infected or reaches sufficient size to cause symptoms. The reason may be incorrect placement or dislocation of the drains, or even too early removal. Occasionally the drains may evoke a reaction of the peritoneal surface of their own and thus further increase the size of, or seal off, the early accumulations. Subhepatic accumulations are the most common of the serious complications following biliary tract surgery and may occur in 5 to 6 per cent of all patients.

The bile in the subhepatic collections may come from a rent in the gallbladder bed or bile ducts. It may be the result of a ligature slipping off the cystic duct or of insecure closure of a choledochotomy. Most often, it comes directly from the liver parenchyma following removal of the gallbladder. The liver is soft and easily damaged during cholecystectomy. Not infrequently, there are bile ductules directly in the bed from which the gallbladder is removed. These are often torn during its removal, especially when the surgeon fails to find the proper plane for dissection. Along with lacerations of the liver substance itself, these tears contribute mainly to the bile collections. Blood and lymph are mixed with the bile in various proportions. The lymph channels in the porta hepatis are abundant, although not always grossly recognizable. Bleeding is usually only a problem when deep lacerations of the liver tissue have occurred or when long-standing damage to the liver has brought on the manifestations of portal hypertension. The symptoms and signs of subhepatic collections may be mild—some right upper quadrant discomfort with tenderness, leukocytosis, and temperature elevation. A more serious picture may develop if frank, purulent infection is present or jaundice

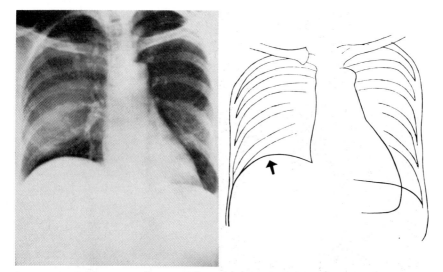

Figure 8–1 Subhepatic collection following cholecystectomy. The patient, a 56 year old woman, was admitted to The New York Hospital–Cornell Medical Center three weeks following a cholecystectomy performed at another hospital. Bleeding during the operation and signs of renewed bleeding during the postoperative course necessitated transfusions. The patient arrived here in severe pain and was anemic, with a palpable right upper quadrant mass. The illustration shows elevation of the right leaf of the diaphragm. (From Thorbjarnarson, B., and Glenn, F.: Complications of biliary tract surgery. Surg. Clin. North Am. *44*:431, 1964.)

supervenes, The jaundice may be from pressure and irritative reaction of the periductal collection or from reflex spasms of the sphincter of Oddi. If infection of the bile has occurred, acute episodes of cholangitis are superimposed. The expanding subhepatic collections may extend in any direction, into the free abdominal cavity or the subphrenic spaces. In these cases, the systemic manifestations become correspondingly aggravated and the indications for surgical drainage all the more prominent.

BILE PERITONITIS

Bile peritonitis occurs when there is leakage of bile from the liver or the extrahepatic biliary tree into the peritoneal cavity. This bile may come from a laceration of the liver tissue, involving large or small bile canaliculi within the parenchyma, or from bile ducts injured or divided in the capsule during removal of the gallbladder. Bile also may escape from the large extrahepatic ducts when a ligature on the cystic duct fails or when injuries to the main duct are not recog-

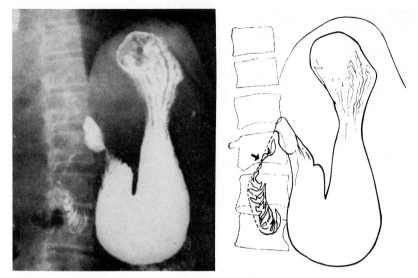

Figure 8–2 Subhepatic collection following cholecystectomy. Same patient as in Figure 8–1. A radiographic study of the stomach and duodenum reveals extrinsic pressure on the second portion of the duodenum. Following transfusions and work-up the patient was explored, and a large infected subhepatic hematoma was evacuated. (From Thorbjarnarson, B., and Glenn, F.: Complications of biliary tract surgery. Surg. Clin. North Am. *44*:431, 1964.)

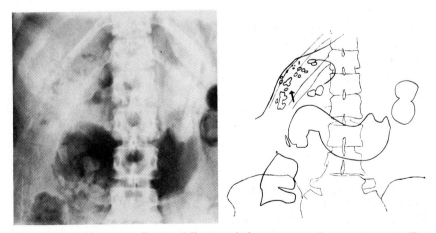

Figure 8–3 Subhepatic collection following cholecystectomy. Same patient as in Figure 8–1. The radiolucent areas in the right upper quadrant, as seen on a scout film of the abdomen, are characteristic of air bubbles in a subhepatic collection. (From Thorbjarnarson, B., and Glenn, F.: Complications of biliary tract surgery. Surg. Clin. North Am. *44*:431, 1964.)

nized during surgery. Bile peritonitis has been known to result from the routine removal of a T-tube following common duct exploration, or from the needle hole in the liver from biopsy or in the wall of the common duct from an intraoperative cholangiogram.

The amount of bile escaping into the abdominal cavity depends on the size of the bile ducts injured and whether distal obstruction is present. After any operation on the biliary tree, it is likely that some degree of obstruction resulting from spasm or swelling around the lower end of the common duct exists, and this tends to divert the bile from its normal passageway. This obstruction is usually self-limited and temporary. When complete division of a bile duct has occurred, of course, all the bile produced by that part of the liver escapes into the peritoneal cavity. Overlooked stones or unrecognized tumors of the pancreas or ampulla of Vater tend to increase the danger of bile peritonitis, unless adequate drainage of the common duct has been provided.

Diagnostic studies in the form of percutaneous liver biopsies are prone, on occasion, to cause escape of bile into the peritoneal cavity. This is particularly so when the patient is suffering from obstructive jaundice or if the gallbladder is perforated.

The signs and symptoms of bile peritonitis vary considerably, and it is hard to define what the classic picture of the entity is. Small amounts of bile have been known to give rise to severe pain and marked systemic reaction; on the other hand, large collections can be found in patients with minimal signs and discomfort. Bile may act as a noxious agent on the serosal surfaces of the abdomen. In these cases enormous amounts of fluid may collect in the abdominal cavity. The large amount of fluid is thought to accumulate from exudation through the damaged peritoneum. The main symptom in such cases is progressive abdominal distention, associated with internal dehydration from loss of intravascular fluid, sunken eyes, poor skin turgor, oliguria, and hemoconcentration. The local signs of peritonitis may be minimal, but usually there is an increase in pulse rate, with mental torpor and lassitude. We have seen patients with bile peritonitis as described above, but we have also seen cases in which the signs of peritonitis predominated. Severe, acute pain is present, spreading all over the abdomen, with radiation to both shoulders and corresponding muscle guarding, but there is no dehydration, hemoconcentration, or rise in the pulse rate. Still we see persons showing a combination of the two pictures, and these persons are often the ones most severely ill.

The treatment of bile peritonitis involves prompt evacuation and adequate drainage. When loss of intravascular fluid into the peritoneal cavity has been severe and oliguria has set in, restoration of the circulating blood volumes is the most important step in addition to drainage. The maintenance of adequate urine output is often difficult and requires constant watching, with hourly determination of urine volume and frequent assessment of hematocrit for evidence of further loss of fluid into the peritoneal cavity or tissue space.

BILIARY FISTULAS

Following operations upon the biliary tract, there is normally slight drainage of bile from the operative area. Usually this drainage diminishes steadily over a period of days and then stops with healing of the wound following removal of the drains. This is true whether drainage has been established by decompression of the biliary tract and drainage of the subhepatic space, such as following common duct exploration, or whether it has been established by drainage of the subhepatic space alone, such as following cholecystectomy. When there is prolonged drainage of bile following removal of the drains and decompression tubes, a biliary fistula exists. When bile peritonitis is discovered at operation, it may be possible to identify the source of leakage and redirect the flow of bile into the intestine or establish adequate drainage to the exterior. In the latter case, a fistula may result.

An established biliary fistula is a serious complication of surgery, which is dangerous to the patient and often difficult for the surgeon to correct. It almost always requires a secondary operation. Still, external fistula is of less immediate danger to the patient than bile peritonitis and allows time and opportunity for the surgeon to make diagnostic studies and prepare the patient for further surgery. Biliary fistulas may occur after any operation on the biliary tract. Following cholecystostomy, there is frequently persistent drainage of mucus and bile from the sinus tract after removal of the drainage tube. Usually this drainage is small and intermittent and is dependent on outflow obstruction in the cystic duct or ampullary portion of the gallbladder.[4] A stone left behind may allow bile to flow into the gallbladder, but it will block the outflow so that, once in the gallbladder, the bile flows more readily to the outside than back to the common duct. This may also occur without residual stones. The treatment for this type of fistula is an elective cholecystectomy. Incomplete cholecystectomy may give rise to a fistula. It is not uncommon, on reoperation for the persistent drainage of bile, to find a remnant of the gallbladder still present, usually containing some calcareous material. Such patients are relieved following removal of the gallbladder remnant and of the cystic duct to within 5 mm of the common duct wall. Other causes of biliary fistula following cholecystectomy include loss of integrity of the wall of the common duct incurred during the operation and obstruction of the duct distal to the cystic duct. The obstruction may be caused by a tumor of the ampulla of Vater, pancreas, or common duct; a residual stone; calcareous material; or a stricture (see Fig. 6–14). Whatever the cause, after a period of obstruction bile escapes from the stump of the cystic duct, with the establishment of a biliary fistula. Obstructive jaundice may thus be the first sign in the development of a fistula and usually indicates a complete obstruction or loss of continuity in the common duct.

The loss of bile sustained by the patient depends on the size and completeness of the fistula. The amount of bile drained in 24 hours gives an indication of how complete the fistula is. Ordinarily an adult person produces from 1000 to 1500 ml of bile in 24 hours. The excretory function of the liver, however, is altered after surgery and after a severe complication. Part of the bile lost into the abdomen is reabsorbed, and drainage to the outside in a complete biliary fistula may only be 500 to 700 ml per 24 hours. The bile lost is rich in electrolytes, and continued loss ultimately depletes the body. It is therefore important to institute replacement therapy as soon as feasible. The simplest form of replacement is to use the bile itself. Collection of the bile from the fistula is sometimes a problem, but we find now that disposable plastic bags glued to the skin around the fistula, on the same principle as ileostomy bags, are most satisfactory. The use of these plastic containers is not feasible when the bile drains out through a large and possibly infected wound. In these cases the insertion of a stump drain attached to a mild suction device may solve the problem. Once the bile is collected, it is strained and stored in a cold place. To feed the bile back to the patient, a small-caliber nasogastric tube may be used; surprisingly enough, many patients have no trouble drinking the bile taking small quantities at a time.

Once the bile is being replaced, the patient usually gains strength, and diagnostic studies may be carried out. Important information may be gained from a review of the surgical procedure that preceded the occurrence of the fistula, but often this information may be difficult to obtain. Among the diagnostic procedures available is injection of radiopaque material into the fistula. This sometimes demonstrates the bile ducts and locates the area of injury or obstruction. Intravenous cholangiography may at times visualize the ductal system. This, combined with radiologic examination of the duodenum, may reveal lesions of the ampulla of Vater or the head of the pancreas. Percutaneous transhepatic cholangiography is rarely of help in accurate preoperative diagnosis of fistula, but a retrograde cholangiogram through a duodenoscope may be of help.

Draining fistulas usually come directly from the biliary tree proper but also may result from disruption of a duodenotomy. The closure of the duodenotomy following transduodenal exploration of the common duct has to be carefully accomplished. Occasionally, insecure closure or factors beyond the surgeon's control lead to disruption of the duodenal wound. Along with the bile, there is drainage of gastric juice and pancreatic enzymes. Because of the activation of the proteolytic enzymes, there is prominent excoriation of the skin and actual digestion of the tissues if adequate protection is not given.

When adequate drainage is established, there is a possibility that duodenal fistulas may heal without further treatment. Replacement of fluid and electrolyte loss and protection of the skin are the two important factors in conservative treatment. Nutritional factors may necessitate jejunostomy for feeding purposes, and occasionally a partial gastrectomy may be advisable to bypass the duodenal segment and facilitate healing. Total intravenous hyperalimentation is now one of the main lines of defense in treatment of intestinal fistulas. The treatment of biliary fistulas thus depends on their etiologic factors. Surgery is usually necessary following diagnostic work-up. Distal common duct obstruction has to be relieved by removal of the stone or resection or bypass of the tumor present. The correct approach to the problem is thus often not obvious until the time of operation, and the surgeon has to be prepared to adapt his therapy to the findings in each case. The implantation of a fistulous tract into bowel as the treatment for biliary fistulas ignores the various factors responsible and usually is unsatisfactory.

HEMORRHAGE

This complication may be found in any large series of patients and may come from several different sources. The bleeding may be due to insufficient hemostasis at operation or to a frank bleeding tendency associated with liver damage and/or lack of vitamin K for prothrombin production. In long-standing biliary tract disease with marked liver damage, a bleeding tendency may be caused by failure of the liver to produce the clotting elements rather than by failure to absorb vitamin K. In these instances there may be little or no response to administration of the vitamin. We use administration of vitamin K and its response as a therapeutic test in evaluating patients for operation. When there is a 20 per cent or more reduction of prothrombin activity with no response to vitamin K administration, it is likely that surgical intervention will be hazardous and probably contraindicated. Bleeding is frequently encountered aside from that caused by derangement of clotting factors. This may be from the liver itself, from the branches of the hepatic or portal veins, or from the cystic artery. Rarely, an injury may occur to the vena cava. Bleeding from the liver itself is much less likely to occur when the operator succeeds in entering the right plane in his dissection and thus manages to leave intact the fibrous capsule covering the gallbladder fossa. When liver tissue is laid bare or lacerated, bleeding may assume serious proportions. Lacerations of the liver during cholecystectomy are more likely to occur in the swollen and engorged liver sometimes seen in people with borderline heart failure or fatty infiltration. Occasionally, the gallbladder becomes avulsed from the liver, if care is not observed, and the results may be disastrous. Portal hypertension, an occasional sequela of long-standing biliary tract disease, may at times play the villain. Bleeding during cholecystectomy in a person with portal hypertension may be quite difficult to control; we feel that, when the presence of portal hypertension is known, cholecystectomy should be avoided whenever possible. Often cholecystostomy may be substituted.

The common and various anomalies of the vascular supply of the liver and biliary tree make it necessary to exercise due caution during surgery. Proper identification of the vessels involved before division or the application of hemostats is a prerequisite. When bleeding occurs, temporary occlusion of the hepatic artery and portal vein by finger pressure on the hepatoduodenal ligament should be employed to allow proper exposure of the vessel involved. The application of hemostats blindly through pools of blood is only likely to aggravate the insult already sustained and perhaps involve other structures as well. The cystic artery is the main vessel to be divided in cholecystectomy. Most often, this artery arises from the common hepatic or the right hepatic artery. The vessel may be short or long. Division or ligation of the right hepatic artery is a possible complication of surgery or of an attempt to stop hemorrhage. The result may be necrosis of the right lobe of the liver, although administration of antibiotics may alleviate the situation.

The signs and symptoms of bleeding following operations on the biliary tree are usually the same as those following operations elsewhere. There is pallor, sweating, restlessness, rapid pulse, and falling blood pressure. When these signs are corrected by the administration of blood, the assumption may be made that bleeding exists, which usually requires reoperation with search for and securing of the source of bleeding. Continuous, slow bleeding may be evidenced by a gradual falling in the person's hematocrit, prolonged oozing of blood from drain sites, or the formation of a mass in the right upper quadrant. The formation of a hematoma of sufficient size for palpation in the right upper quadrant requires evacuation and better drainage, since absorption of blood is slow and the danger of secondary infection from the bile considerable.

COMPLICATIONS ASSOCIATED WITH THE USE
OF DRAINAGE TUBES

Obstruction Due to Occluded Tubes

Drainage tubes in the common duct necessarily encroach upon its lumen. Any deposit inside these tubes increases the obstruction first in the tube and later in the duct itself. The duct has a remarkable capacity for dilation, and complete obstruction therefore seldom occurs. As time goes by, however, encrustations and deposits from the bile accumulate and increase in size. In the early postoperative period, such deposits or blood clots may be flushed out easily by gentle irrigation of the tube, using saline or water. Later this becomes more and more difficult, and ultimately such tubes have to be removed. There is great variation in how long tubes remain patent in the biliary tree. We have seen some function adequately for 15 years, whereas others have to be removed within months. Use of solvent or irrigating fluid other than saline or water is not recommended.[3]

Retention of Drainage Tubes

Occasionally, difficulty is encountered in removing drainage tubes from the common duct. This may be due to both a suture securing the tube to the duct and closure of the duct around the tube, which should be bile-tight. When fine catgut is used for these sutures, it should not be difficult to remove the tube about ten days following operation. When the tube is not removed readily on the first try, it is better to desist and try again later. It may be helpful to apply traction to the tube, then set a clamp across it at skin level and have the patient walk about. The maintenance of continuous mild traction often succeeds in dislodging the tube. When large T-tubes of fairly stiff rubber are used, it is helpful to cut a V-shaped piece out of the tube opposite the external limb. This segment may include up to half the circumference of the tube and allow it to buckle more easily on removal.

Dislocation of Drainage Tubes

Following common duct exploration, the duct should be drained and decompressed by the use of a T-tube or a straight catheter emerging from the cystic duct. The tube may occasionally become dislocated; it may be caught in the dressings and thus removed when these are changed, or it may be anchored to the bed or the sheets and be pulled out when the patient sits up or turns around in bed. If adequate slack is not afforded when the tube is placed at operation, it may be partly dislocated when the patient wakes up and recovers his muscle tone. The patient may pick at and possibly remove the tube during recovery from anesthesia. To avoid this, care should be taken during the operation to leave some slack on the tube intra-abdominally. The tube may be secured to the duct with a suture and should also be attached to the skin with a silk suture. The suture securing the tube to the bile duct should be of fine catgut, which will not interfere with later removal. As the tube emerges from the skin, it may be secured over a roll of gauze, which again is attached by adhesive to the skin separately from the main dressings. The patient should also be instructed as to the function of the tube, so that he will be on guard against inadvertent dislocation or removal.

When a tube becomes dislocated shortly after the operation, a serious situation may develop. Possibly the escape of bile will be small and insignificant; then it is usually best to allow the dislocated tube to remain inside the abdomen, since it may provide a tract for escape of bile to the outside. The drains which are placed at the foramen of Winslow and which emerge along the gallbladder fossa to the outside also may be sufficient to evacuate any bile that escapes. When there is distal obstruction, there is usually an escape of large amounts of bile. These patients may develop signs of bile peritonitis and should be carefully observed for immediate exploration and drainage should this develop. The length of the tubes inside the bile duct is important. A tube that extends far into the lower part of the duct may both occlude the outflow of bile and be occluded itself from the end resting against the wall of the duct. In both instances, bile leakage around the tube will occur. A tube that extends too far into the hepatic duct may only drain one side of the liver and possibly interfere with drainage from the other lobe. The T-tubes used for the routine drainage of the bile duct should be the smallest caliber to give adequate drainage, and the limbs inside the duct should be short enough not to extend to the end of the common or hepatic ducts. A biliary fistula based on a T-tube blocking the lower end of the duct may be diagnosed by x-ray study. Usually the duct dilates and allows flow around the tube into the duodenum, but on odd occasions the tube has to be removed to cure the problem.

JAUNDICE FOLLOWING OPERATIONS UPON THE BILIARY TRACT

Calculi and Strictures

Calculi and strictures are the most common cause of jaundice following biliary tract operations.[1,8] If cholecystostomy or common duct exploration has been carried out, the onset of jaundice should not be expected until the tubes have been removed and the tract to the outside has healed. We customarily determine the common duct pressures and obtain a cholangiogram before removing the drainage tubes. We expect the ductal pressures to be 30 cm of water or less. Cholangiography is performed, usually on the tenth or eleventh day following operation. The radiograph should demonstrate all the main branches of the bile duct without defects and free flow of dye into the duodenum. When stones or obstructing lesions are demonstrated, the tube should not be removed until surgical correction has been carried out. Stones may be left behind in the ductal system during chole-cystostomy or cholecystectomy with or without choledochotomy. When unsuspected stones are overlooked, they may become sympto-matic, and when suspected stones are not detected, the symptoms are usually aggravated following the operation.

The onset of right quadrant pain associated with some fever and jaundice following cholecystectomy, especially when the pain is brought on and worsened by feeding, is almost pathognomonic for retained common duct stone. When the jaundice is mild or evanes-cent, the diagnosis usually can be established by intravenous chol-

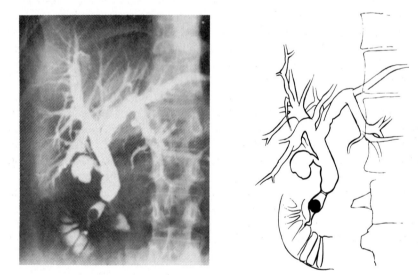

Figure 8–4   Jaundice following an operation on the biliary tree. A 65 year old woman was admitted to The New York Hospital–Cornell Medical Center. An operation had been performed six months previously at another hospital. A diagnosis of carcinoma of the gallbladder had been made without histologic corroboration, and a course of radiation therapy had been given. The patient was jaundiced on admission here. The percutaneous cholangiogram shows a stone in the lower end of the common duct. This was confirmed at the operation which followed. There was no evidence of tumor. (From Thorbjarnarson, B., and Glenn, F.: Complications of biliary tract surgery. Surg. Clin. North Am. 44:431, 1964.)

angiography.[5] When the jaundice deepens and is protracted, percutaneous cholangiography usually is successful in outlining the obstruction.[2]

The reason why stones tend to become symptomatic following operations is not obvious. Incision, instrumentation, and repair of the common duct during operation undoubtedly cause some spasm, swelling, and edema. Spasm of the musculature of the sphincter of Oddi resulting from trauma probably leads to impaction of the offending stone.

After the functioning gallbladder is removed, the common duct usually enlarges. There is also a change in the hydrodynamics of the duct, since bile now tends to flow directly into the duodenum, because the intermediate reservoir has been removed. This may allow stones to drop into the lower reaches of the common duct, where impaction followed by obstruction is more likely to occur. Since common duct stones tend to increase in incidence with age, investigation of the duct should be undertaken more often in the elderly than in the young. Intravenous cholangiography preoperatively should materially aid in detecting common duct stones. The cholangiograms may reveal the stone or show dilatation of the duct alone in intraoperative cholangiography.

Malignant Tumors

Next to calculi, malignant tumors are the most common cause of obstructive jaundice, When the removal of an acalculous gallbladder is followed by jaundice, the suspicion is reinforced, since the combination of common duct stones and an acalculous gallbladder is distinctly rare. The findings at operation in the early phase of malignant obstruction to the lower end of the common duct may be equivocal. Ordinarily, however, the common duct is dilated and thin-walled even before the onset of jaundice, and the same may be true for the gallbladder. When exploration of the dilated common duct does not reveal stones but there is still difficulty in demonstrating patency of the choledochoduodenal junction, transduodenal exposure of the ampulla of Vater is essential to elucidate the diagnosis. Calculi and carcinoma of the ampulla of Vater or pancreas are not common together, but when this occurs, it may be difficult to establish the correct diagnosis. Pancreatitis from biliary tract disease may easily mimic carcinoma and vice versa, and biopsies at the time of operation are not likely to be conclusive. Ampullary carcinoma can often be detected by transduodenal exploration, but the same is not true for pancreatic cancer.

Pancreatitis

Pancreatitis is commonly associated with calculous biliary tract disease. As a rule, the pancreatic involvement subsides following removal of the calculous gallbladder or common duct stones. Once in a while, an exacerbation of pancreatitis follows biliary tract surgery, and rarely this may be severe enough to cause obstructive jaundice. Manipulation of the pancreas or forceful dilatation of the sphincter of Oddi with resultant trauma to the pancreatic duct may be responsible. Pancreatitis is particularly feared by some surgeons following operations on the sphincter of Oddi. It is our belief that this complication should not happen too often when proper precautions are taken during surgery. The treatment of postoperative pancreatitis is conservative and involves institution of nasogastric suction and administration of antibiotics, along with electrolyte and volume replacement. The use of vagolytic agents is debatable, since in sufficient dosage they also aggravate existing ileus or bring it on and may add urinary retention to the patient's problems. Only rarely will reoperation for common duct drainage be necessary, unless a residual stone has complicated the picture.

Cholangitis — Chronic Liver Damage

Acute cholangitis is seldom a problem postoperatively when adequate common duct decompression has been carried out. Forceful irrigation of common duct drainage tubes is contraindicated because it may be followed by a flare-up in intraductal infection. We have observed this subsequent to postoperative cholangiography. During the procedure the patient usually experiences some pain followed by a chill. The causes are the irritating action of the contrast material, the forcefulness of the injection, and the presence of bacteria in the biliary tree. When fever follows cholangiography, the drainage tube should be left open and should not be removed until resolution has occurred. Occasionally antibiotics may be required.

Some patients with long-standing biliary tract disease have a markedly diminished liver reserve, although this may not be obvious by routine preoperative investigation. This is especially true when multiple common duct stones or deposits of sand fill the ductal system. These patients may have only minimal symptoms, but for years the bile has been filtered through the stone deposits, which causes a certain amount of back pressure on the liver parenchyma. Low-grade infection is also present, and because of structural changes in the walls of the bile ducts, it is difficult to eradicate. Jaundice may occur here but is rarely severe, although it may occasionally be progressive. The patients often are listless, with loss of energy and appetite. Their course is tedious and prolonged. Recovery is based on affording adequate nutrition to allow the liver time and opportunity for recovery. Eradication of intraductal infection by antibiotic therapy facilitates the reparative process.

Incompatible Transfusions — Viral Hepatitis

Among the rare causes of jaundice following biliary tract surgery, but not peculiar to it, are the administration of incompatible blood and viral hepatitis. When incompatible blood is given, hemolysis is the result, often accompanied by renal failure. The jaundice in itself is not the major problem; the renal impairment constitutes the actual danger to the patient. Viral hepatitis following biliary tract surgery usually manifests itself in liver function tests, indicating parenchymal rather than obstructive jaundice. Usually hepatitis is contracted by serum or blood administration but may also have been transmitted in another way. Anesthetic agents have been implicated in liver damage and jaundice after operations. Halothane hepatitis, real or not, has been reported, and many anesthesiologists avoid its use in patients with biliary disease.

Metastatic Carcinoma

Occasionally patients are seen with obstructive jaundice following biliary tract surgery, and re-exploration reveals metastatic carcinoma in the liver as the cause. A further search may reveal a primary tumor elsewhere in the gastrointestinal tract that has been overlooked as the source of the metastasis. Occasionally, however, no primary tumor is found on re-exploration, but a review of the previous operation and the tissue removed brings to light a carcinoma of the gallbladder, which in the meantime has spread diffusely throughout the liver.

INFECTION

The bile in normal individuals ordinarily is sterile. Under usual conditions the biliary tract clears itself of bacteria that pass through the liver, and only when inflammatory response is created in the gallbladder or in the ductal wall do the bacteria remain as pathogenic organisms within the biliary tract. Once stones are present within the biliary tract, damage occurs to the mucosa, and bacteria carried to the biliary tree through the lymphatics and blood supply of the liver become inhabitants of the biliary tree. The longer these conditions prevail, the higher is the incidence of bacteria isolated from the bile, the stones within the biliary tree, or the wall of the biliary tree.

Infection has always played a major role in the complications of biliary tract surgery and has always been a major source of complications and even death in patients suffering from biliary tract disease with or without operative intervention. The most common causes of death following biliary tract surgery today are afflictions of the cardiovascular system. Even though the causes of death are listed as cardiovascular, the death is usually preceded by some septic or infectious complication which is a major contributor to the patient's death.

Use of Antibiotics

The control of biliary tract infection is accomplished both by timely surgery and by appropriate and judicious use of antibiotics. The average healthy patient undergoing surgery for uncomplicated gallbladder diseases does not need antibiotic treatment, but an integral part of surgery for any type of biliary tract disease should be culture of the bile in the gallbladder or from the cystic duct stump at the time of surgery. The surgeon will receive reports on bacteria growth and sensitivity studies from these maneuvers within a few days after surgery and can therefore be prepared for the antibiotic treatment of any septic complication that might arise, since wound infections or intra-abdominal abscesses following biliary tract surgery usually contain the same organisms that are cultured from the bile at the time of the primary surgery. The most common organisms found in the bile or in the wall of the gallbladder are *E. coli*, staphylococci, *Klebsiella* A-type bacteria, and clostridia.[9-12] A wide variety of different organisms can be found, but these four types of organisms are responsible for over 80 per cent of positive cultures from the biliary tract. It has become evident from numerous studies that particular groups of patients are more apt to have biliary bacteremia than others and are thus more likely to develop some other septic complications associated with biliary tract disease or surgery.[12] These patients have been identified as those having acute cholecystitis, those with common duct stones and obstructive jaundice, and old people, particularly over the age of 70. A very high percentage of these patients are found to have bacteria in the bile at the time of surgery, and the incidence of septic complications is greatly increased among them. It has therefore become clear that this group of patients might benefit more than others from protective coverage by judiciously applied antibiotics.

There has been controversy surrounding the value of antibiotics in the treatment of cholecystitis, particularly since in acute cholecystitis bacteria within the gallbladder are hardly accessible to the systemically administered antibiotics, since the cystic duct is obstructed and the antibiotics can only reach the bile through the wall of the gallbladder. It has also become evident that preoperatively administered antibiotics in biliary tract surgery do not lessen the biliary bacteremia, as defined by positive cultures obtained at surgery.[10] It has been found, however, that antibiotics administered immediately preoperatively and for a short period postoperatively have materially diminished the occurrence of septic complications postoperatively. This is explained by the action of the antibiotics in the tissues surrounding the gallbladder and the biliary tree and by their effects on bacteria in these locations rather than in the biliary tract itself, where the infection originated. On the basis of present information, it would seem advisable to administer antibiotics immediately preoperatively and also postoperatively to patients in the categories mentioned earlier who are undergoing biliary tract surgery.

The type of antibiotics used will vary from time to time, depending on patterns of existence developed. In a recent study it was demonstrated that, although both ampicillin and loridine were found to be effective, there was a higher number of bacteria resistant to ampicillin than to luridine, as determined by cultures done at the time of the operation. The choice of type of antibiotic to be administered will have to take into account possible allergies on the part of the patient. The antibiotics should also be able to affect both gram-positive and gram-negative bacteria. Cultures taken at surgery or through blood cultures obtained prior to surgery will guide the way to more proper administration of antibiotics for the individual patient. I have been using ampicillin, unless otherwise indicated, in doses of 1 g intravenously four times a day, with the first dose given during surgery, unless it is started earlier as indicated by the clinical status of the patient prior to surgery.

REFERENCES

1. Cattell, R. B., and Braasch, J.: Primary repair of benign strictures of the bile ducts. Surg. Gynecol. Obstet. 109:531, 1959.
2. Glenn, F., Evans, J. A., Mujahed, Z., and Thorbjarnarson, B.: Percutaneous transhepatic cholangiography. Ann. Surg. 156:451, 1962.

3. Glenn, F.: Management of common duct drainage. Surg. Gynecol. Obstet. *105*:238, 1957.
4. Glenn, F.: Importance of technique in cholecystectomy. Surg. Gynecol. Obstet. *101*:201, 1955.
5. Johnson, G., Pearce, C., and Glenn, F.: Intravenous cholangiography in biliary tract disease. Ann. Surg. *152*:91, 1960.
6. Sims, J. M.: Remarks on cholecystostomy in dropsy of the gallbladder. Br. Med. J. June 8, 1878, p. 811.
7. Thorbjarnarson, B., and Glenn, F.: Complications of biliary tract surgery. Surg. Clin. North Am. *44*:431, 1964.
8. Walters, W., Nixon, J. W., Jr., and Hodgins, T. E.: Strictures of the common bile duct: Five to 25 year follow-up of 217 operations. Ann. Surg. *149*:781, 1959.
9. Chetlin, S. H., and Elliott, D. W.: Preoperative antibiotics in biliary surgery. Arch. Surg. *107*:319, 1973.
10. Chetlin, S. H., and Elliott, D. W.: Biliary bacteremia. Arch. Surg. *102*:303, 1971.
11. Fukunaga, F. H.: Gallbladder bacteriology, histology and gallstones. Arch. Surg. *106*:169, 1973.
12. Mason, G. R.: Bacteriology and antibiotic selection in biliary tract surgery. Arch. Surg. *97*:533, 1968.

Index

Note: Page numbers in *italics* refer to illustrations.

163

165